P9-DZZ-916

A BEGINNER'S GUIDE TO ESSENTIAL OILS

Recipes and Practices for a Natural Lifestyle and Holistic Health

By

Hayley Hobson

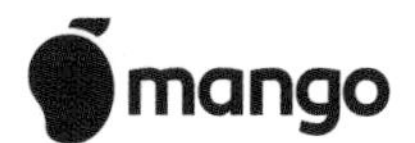

Published by Mango Publishing Group, a division of Mango Media Inc.

Cover, Design & Layout: Morgane Leoni

For permission requests, please contact the publisher at:

Mango Publishing Group
2850 Douglas Road, 3rd Floor
Coral Gables, FL 33134 U.S.A.
info@mango.bz

For special orders, quantity sales, course adoptions and corporate sales, please email the publisher at sales@mango.bz. For trade and wholesale sales, please contact Ingram Publisher Services at customer.service@ingramcontent.com or +1.800.509.4887.

A BEGINNER'S GUIDE TO ESSENTIAL OILS: Recipes and Practices for a Natural Lifestyle and Holistic Health

Library of Congress Cataloging
ISBN: (p) 978-1-63353-700-2, (e) 978-1-63353-701-9
Library of Congress Control Number: 2017959459
BISAC - HEA011000 HEALTH & FITNESS / Herbal Medications
- HEA016000 HEALTH & FITNESS / Naturopathy HEA032000
- HEALTH & FITNESS / Alternative Therapies

Printed in the United States of America

Table of Contents

INTRODUCTION

A Beginner's Guide to Essential Oils

WELCOME TO the world of essential oils, friend! I love introducing essential oils to novices because it gives me the opportunity to pass along information that will help you make educated choices about the quality and specific oils to meet your needs.

Every time you chop herbs for your salad or sprinkle cinnamon on your oatmeal, you get to experience essential oil compounds. They are concentrated aromatic liquids. Pour a cup of chamomile tea and yep, you do the same. The fragrance and taste can be invigorating, but did you know there are also health benefits?

Essential oils are not a modern discovery. Human culture has been using them for thousands of years. There are tons of varieties and each has special properties.

Ancient Greeks and Romans used essential oils in baths and for rituals. The Chinese and Indians have a long history with oils. Although they were all heavily into aromatic and medicinal use, they also recognized essential oils' ability to influence human feelings.

What You See is Not Always What You Get

What differentiates each essential oil from another? The composition of each oil is what makes it unique, and there are even differences within the same species of botanicals. Quality can be influenced by variations in the production process. My goal is to teach you how and what to look for before you purchase, and what the uses are so you can choose the appropriate oils.

Most people have heard of essential oils and a huge percentage use them daily. The company I purchase my oils from and now partner with enjoys a 68 percent retention rate after people try them and buy them month after month. There are certainly several books on essential oils on the market and lots of information on the Internet. Why, then, would we need another book? Hasn't *this story* been told?

Nope. Not my version!

Since this book is a beginners' guide to essential oils, I'm going to assume you might be right there, you know, at the beginning. Throughout these pages I will introduce you to essential oils and how they can compliment a healthy lifestyle.

I take a holistic approach to present a big picture overview because I want you to get more than what you came for. If I hit on elements you're already familiar with, hang in here with me. It's important to me that my book is comprehensive so true beginners can grow, chapter by chapter.

A Beginner's Guide to Essential Oils is not a textbook, and it's more than a how-to book for using essential oils. Along with education, I share my favorite recipes and blends and easy-to-learn practices you can incorporate immediately. Over the next few chapters, I address personal development and aspects of mental and emotional wellness. Mind and body are connected, and essential oils can benefit both at the same time.

Honestly, if this guide were only about how to choose and use essential oils, it would miss the mark. You see, essential oils are so much more than yummy smelling drops we rub onto pulse points to make us feel better.

Essential oils saved my life.

See, there was a time my life was a hot mess. To say I was under pressure would be an understatement. But as tense as it was, I didn't walk away from my challenges or allow my slips and falls to break my stride. It was just the opposite. I tried even harder.

Some of my most painful lessons became stepping stones to my dreams come true. I believe that in telling my story and teaching my wellness strategies I will reach others, like you, who seek a life of balance. No matter where you are on the wellness scale, there is hope in living a holistic lifestyle.

Wellness isn't just about working on a single aspect of life, like eating or exercise. It is a culmination of all the choices we make in every area: emotional, mental, physical and spiritual. There are essential oils to support each of these. How do I know? Because I've experienced it. I began using oils and have never stopped. I still use them every day.

I'm going to walk this path beside you as you learn ways to integrate powerful wellness modalities with essential oils. My desire is to support you in living the life you've only dreamed about.

So, let's begin our journey.

Chapter One

My Story

I'M NOT exaggerating when I say that several years ago, incorporating essential oils as part of my wellness program saved my life. I was virtually one breath away from the edge and the only thing left was for me to take that final step. But I never gave up.

My body was deteriorating. It was responding to a noxious lifestyle and mental state; neither of which were very healthy. I had been dealing with poor health since I was a child and it was coming to a head.

Here's where my story began.

At the age of five, I was diagnosed with severe stomach issues, starting a chain reaction of illness that continued until I was forty years old. My health eventually got so bad that my liver, pancreas and other organs started shutting down—I was experiencing autoimmune disease-like symptoms. Can you imagine living this way as an adult, let alone as a child?

My dad was a doctor and what kid doesn't hang on every word their dad says? He was compassionate with my health challenges and really tried to help. He believed western Medicine had all the answers, and I trusted it because he did. We never questioned it, even though I wasn't getting well.

Throughout my young life and into adulthood, I ended up in the hospital for weeks at a time, on IV antibiotics. This weakened my immune system and irritated my gut even more. It had also probably been irritated from the toxic products and foods *my* body could not digest. So, basically, I had a stomach ache my entire life.

As most of society at the time, we didn't know what we didn't know. We consumed too much dairy, and I later found out I was completely lactose intolerant. We used household cleaning and personal care products that today head the list of contributors to sickness and disease. Most of the western world didn't know wellness was in our own hands and so we lived toxic lives.

People who know me are shocked to hear that when I was young I was super insecure and gawky. I wasn't just shy. I was petrified; literally unable to hold a conversation.

In high school and college, I was terrified in social situations, and as an adult I used to have to hold a drink in my hand just to relax. My insecurity was serious.

I finished college and went to law school. After passing the bar I opened a law practice within a boutique firm and I was pretty successful, earning a six-figure income. Most people in my position would have been happy. But I wasn't.

You see, I didn't want to be a lawyer. I followed someone else's plan for my life. I was sad and dissatisfied most of the time, just going through the motions.

Physically, I was a mess; suffering from poor digestion and hardly eating because of it. Seriously, I almost never felt well. Add this to my emotional distress and there wasn't much quality of life. It had been that way for a long time.

I wouldn't go to parties or clubs without heading straight to the bar the minute I walked through the door. OMG! Even to speak to one person freaked me out. I never thought I had anything important to say. So of course, with that kind of thought process, I'd feel nervous just having to open my mouth. I went on that way for many years until one day I found myself at a crossroads. It hit me like a slap in the face.

It was obvious. What I was doing wasn't working and I had run out of road. Two choices were in front of me and I had to make one of them.

Either I could take an honest look at my life and where I was headed, you know, contemplate.

Or I could STOP immediately, own-up to the past choices I had made, turn and walk in another direction.

I chose the latter. If I hadn't, I wouldn't have written this book. Honestly, I am not sure I would even be here today.

I did one of the hardest things any of us can do, and that is to admit I needed to leave behind everything I stood on my entire life. An obsolete thought process and toxic lifestyle were slowly destroying me every single day. I had to acknowledge that what I was doing wasn't working and then make some changes.

It took a lot of courage to act on my new choices for life, but let me tell you, I was ready. I am forever grateful to the part of me that picked me up by the shoulders and set me on my current path; one that embraces Integrative Wellness. That meant looking at the role lifestyle was playing in my health.

If you've ever had to make huge changes in your life, you know that any kind of change requires willingness to be honest with yourself, right? So, what did I do? I opened my mind. I began exploring edgy wellness ideas that went in the opposite direction of the conservative western practices I was raised with.

Along the way, I discovered essential oils, almost by accident. And you know what? I experienced results almost immediately. The oils not only helped support a healthy immune system but also aided in transforming my mental and emotional life.

Do I still suffer from shyness? Not any more. Oh, I still have a moment once in a while, but it feels more like a jolt of adrenaline now. My new thoughts are, "People like me and like what I have to say," and "People want to hear what I have to say." And those kinds of thoughts make me feel WAY more confident.

I'm super grateful that I now feel comfortable in social settings. Want to know the irony? By teaching other people what they have to share matters, I've learned the importance of stepping forward in my own life.

Where Do Essential Oils Come From?

Essential oils come from naturally occurring aromatic liquid found in flowers and plants. You might be surprised to know they also come from tree bark, seeds, roots and other parts of plants. When you bend to smell a Rose, you are taking in the sweet fragrance of its essential oils. Crush some fresh Basil between your fingers and essential oils are released. That smell of pine when walking through a forest? Yep, essential oils.

You might be thinking there must be hundreds of scents. Well, guess what? Over 3,000 essential oils have been identified. Each has its purpose and direct benefit.

In addition to using essential oils to proactively boost your immune and digestive system, they can help balance your hormones. That's right! This is super important because a state of balance can help keep you from reacting to life or freaking out when you're under pressure.

Using essential oils in beauty treatments and for cooking is not a new discovery. For over 6,000 years, various civilizations have made use of them. We still use some of those ancient methods today.

There are lots of recipes that combine different oils for specific purposes. But before you go fishing on the Internet, please wait until you learn how to choose high-quality oils. I'll tell you what to look for, and of course, I've also picked out some awesome blends for you. They're in the back of the book.

My Relationship with Essential Oils

Essential oils are gifts from the earth. Using them has changed my life in so many ways. By learning about their true potential, I discovered my own.

I told you I first discovered the value of essential oils by accident, but I would actually call it serendipity. Once I experienced the changes that came from using essential oils, I felt compelled to share them with others, and so I shifted gears professionally and started teaching people about how to better their quality of life. At the time of this writing, I'm happy to say I've built a strong business helping many thousands of people by introducing them to essential oils.

When I first started, I had nothing to invest in my business except me. Well, that's what happens when you walk away from a six-figure annual income. There I was—no skills, no network, and no budget—nothing but a desire to help other people who, like me, wanted to live toxin-free lives. So, I stepped onto the first wrung of the ladder and began my climb.

Even though money is not first on my list of importance, I believe it's more than okay to earn money—to prosper doing something you love. So, I worked at building my business. Yeah, it was hard work and took time, but at the same time the essential oils sold themselves.

Today, I have a successful business promoting wellness and the use of essential oils. I believe they can be a critical part of a holistic regimen that among other things includes a healthy diet and exercise.

Anyone who knows me knows essential oils are a big part of my life. I use them to help me relax and also to energize.

Truth? You want to know what I love most about my oils? They allow me to navigate the massive amount of chaos going on around me. I'm a momtrepreneur, which means I have a family as well as a business to run. Both need my attention—sometimes at once.

I take my oils with me wherever I go. I fit as many oils as I can fit in my purse and then pack them when I travel. Everyone in my family, all the way down to my eight-year-old daughter, uses essential oils.

As you read through these chapters, remember that wellness requires maintaining lifestyle practices that support it. Everything works together—attitude, oils, diet, exercise, meditation—all of it. How can you incorporate essential oils into your lifestyle? I have a few ideas for you. Chapter two is on the way.

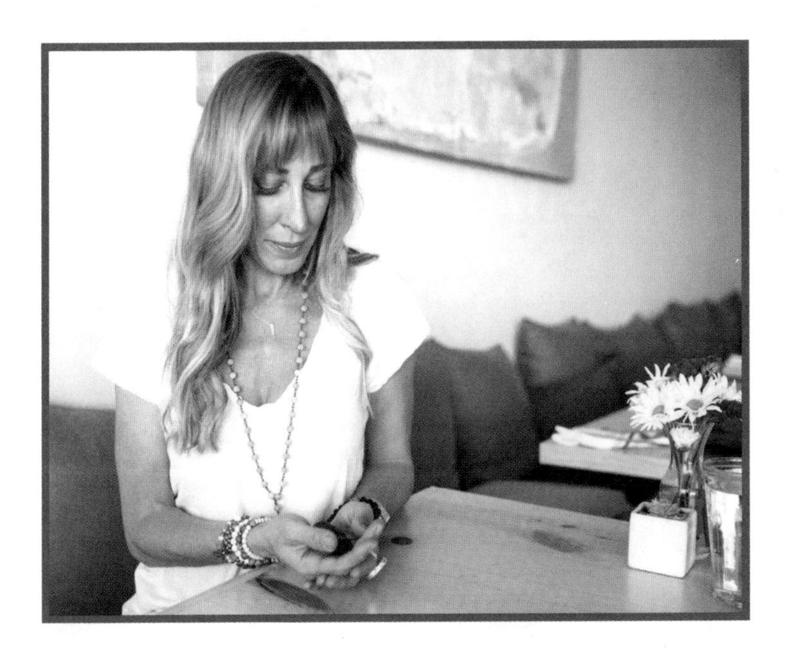

Chapter Two

What Are Essential Oils and How Do You Use Them?

OPEN ANY wellness magazine and you're likely to see something about essential oils. Articles, ads, or uses—lots of people have something to say. It seems essential oils have been the flavor of the decade for professionals on the wellness circuit. The truth is, as I mentioned in the introduction, people have been using them for thousands of years. Everybody has just upped their games and that's why you hear so much about essential oils these days.

Let's review a few key points. Then we'll dig a little deeper into essential oils and how you use them, okay?

In addition to using essential oils as part of a lifestyle to proactively boost your immune and digestive systems, they can help balance your hormones and keep you from freaking out under pressure. You can also have fun with them. Essential oils can be incorporated in beauty treatments and in cooking. They can be used one at a time, or blended for specific purposes.

How to Use Essential Oils

If you're just getting started with essential oils, you might not know all the ways you can use them and what you might use them for. It's easy to feel intimidated when you're learning something new, but the truth is, once you learn, using essential oils is easy. Some methods are more popular than others, and as you work with your oils you'll determine your own habits.

One thing to keep in mind, even though essential oils are safe and non-toxic, you'll want to pay special attention to the guidelines for using certain oils. Some can be taken internally and others only topically. Be sure you don't mix them up.

Even though the scents of some oils are amazing, others might not appeal to you. They're not like perfume although you may enjoy some as personal fragrances. But as I've mentioned, each essential oil has a purpose.

Where to Apply Oils

A popular way to use essential oils is to apply them directly to the skin. Oils are immediately absorbed into your skin because they are fat-soluble. Remember never to apply full-strength. Using more doesn't make an oil work better. Always dilute them with something like fractionated coconut oil. It's wasteful to use more than you need and depending on the oil, that can be expensive.

Dilute with Carrier Oils

Fractionated coconut oil is one of several carrier oils, or base oils, you can use to mix with your essential oils. Dilution is especially important if you have sensitive skin. Carrier oils don't evaporate like essential oils do. But they can go rancid, so be sure the carrier oil you use is fresh.

Apply essential oils to pulse points, such as your wrists. Place a few drops on your palms, rub together and then breathe deeply. And believe it or not, applying oils to your feet is not only popular, but also effective. Your big toe is an especially good spot because it links directly to your brain. You can also choose to apply essential oils on your temples, at the base of your neck or skull, and behind your ears. Apply a few drops of essential oils, inhale, and enjoy.

Begin with a single drop of any oil you're trying for the first time. Make sure you don't have a reaction before you increase to three to four drops. Take any known allergies into consideration before you use the oils.

You'll soon discover that you enjoy some scents more than others, but remember it's not just about the fragrance. It's about the benefits.

Use an Electronic Diffuser

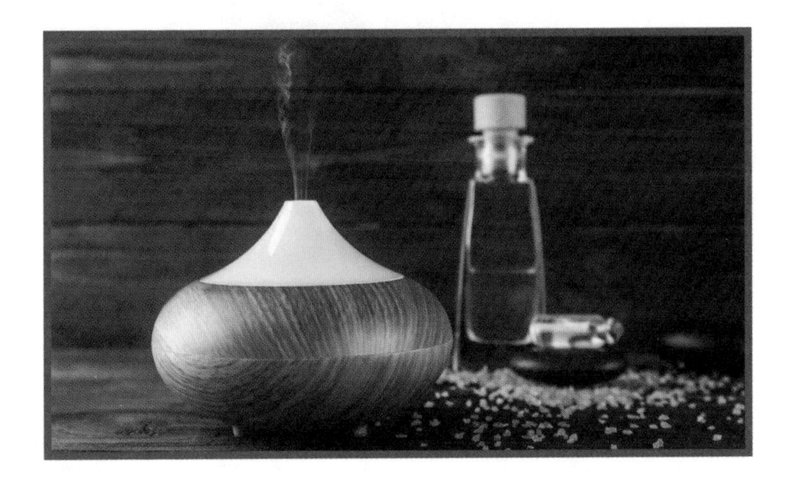

Okay, so THIS is addictive! Plug in your diffuser and a fine mist of essential oils and water sprays, filling the air with the aroma of whatever oil, or combination of oils you use. As the mist circulates, not only will the room smell luscious, but the oils' benefits will also surround you.

There are several types of diffusers. Choose one or two and put one in every room if you like! They are great as gifts, too. I've listed the most popular ones later in the book.

Old-Fashioned Steam

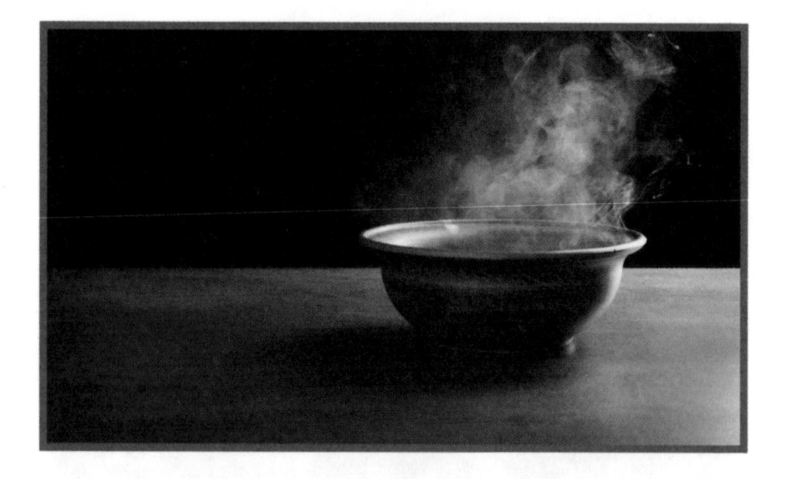

Boil some water and pour into a glass bowl. A few cups will be fine. Add three to four drops of oil to the water and lean in. Cover your head and the bowl with a towel and inhale the steam. You won't have to get too close. Hold your head about eight to twelve inches from the water and breathe in gently and slowly. If you notice any discomfort, stop immediately. You might be allergic.

Aromatherapy Bath

Adding essential oils to your bath is relaxing. Roman Chamomile and Lavender are good choices for a relaxing bath.

Again, don't use them full-strength because they won't dissolve as nicely as they would if you use Epsom salts as a base. Don't use with chemical products!

Another safe, effective way to use essential oils in your bath is to mix them with a carrier oil or milk. The carrier oil will protect your skin from potential irritation and the essential oils bond with the fatty acids in whole milk. Try Rose or Jasmine and milk.

Lavender is calming and nice for a relaxing bath. Add a few drops to soak away stress and tension. If taken internally, Lavender can also reduce anxious feelings. After your bath, take Lavender internally for a peaceful sleep.

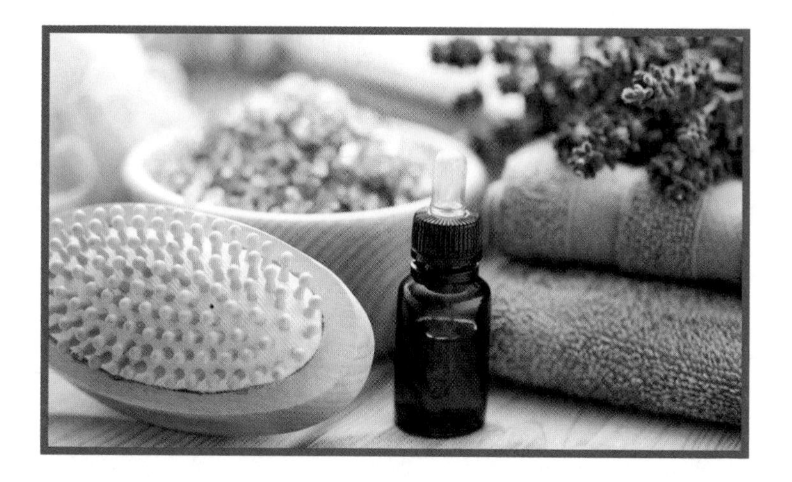

Is MORE Better?

You might really like the scent or flavor of a certain oil, or the benefit of another, but if you think more is better it is not. Essential oils are concentrated. A few drops are plenty and anything more will just be wasted. You might also be sensitive, and some oils cause skin irritation.

In Chapter Eleven, I share some of my favorite essential oil blends. I use them in my own home to keep my family healthy and toxin-free. I encourage you to try them for yourself and your family, to create a healthy, whole and balanced home. Keep reading!

Chapter Three

Essential Oils for Life Balance

I'M A momtrepreneur. I know, crazy word, right? What the heck is a momtrepreneur? It's a funky made-up word that describes an entrepreneur doing the ultimate juggling act—balancing it with life as a mom.

Momtrepreneurs (and entrepreneurs) take risks by investing in their ideas and building businesses. You might be thinking, "Hey, that sounds like fun! I'll quit my job and make money doing something I like for a change! *Piece 'a cake*!"

It is fun, but believe me, life as an entrepreneur is anything but easy. There are no guarantees of success, and there can be a lot of obstacles. When the entrepreneur is a momtrepreneur—the road can be even rockier.

Most momtrepreneurs, myself included, agree that between their families and their businesses there isn't much wiggle room. Our days are jam-packed to say the least. If it were not for my oils I don't know how I'd do it.

This momtrepreneur has two beautiful daughters, and a husband I love spending time with. I lead a super busy life managing my home in Boulder, CO, a beach house in San Diego county, and a successful business with a seven-figure annual income—oftentimes from my phone. Yeah, my phone. It's my office away from home.

I launched my business with the support of my online business plan, including social media strategies, and I created a system to help me balance my life. *Ha!* Or so I thought.

As it turned out, I did just the opposite. Oh, don't get me wrong. For a while, it worked like magic. I got a lot done and my business swelled because of it. I had no complaints. To the contrary, I was jazzed, generating more income than I ever dreamed possible in a surprisingly short time. In less than a year and a half, my customers and business partners were in twenty countries. Today it's over sixty!

Sounds like I created a perfect world for myself, doesn't it? In many ways, yes, I did. But something else also happened.

The more my business grew, the heavier my workload got. Part of my "busyness" came out of the thrill of watching my initial investment snowball. It seemed everything I touched was turning to gold, and so I kept...*touching.*

I've already told you I live a healthy lifestyle. I eat well, a vegan diet, to be exact. I exercise, and I practice Yoga. Juicing is one of my passions. I have a ton of energy, but at one point not too long ago I realized I was wearing myself out. Did I stop running myself ragged? Not at first.

Instead of using my free time to rest or spend with my family, I worked longer hours. The more I got done, the more I added to my plate. About three years into my business, I hit upon a realization that pretty much shocked me. I didn't want to believe it at first, but after a while there was no denying it.

I was addicted. Not to drugs or alcohol, and not directly to my work. I was addicted to the technology that was supposed to free me to live the lifestyle my income level should afford. The gadgets and devices, the apps and software, all imprisoned me. I felt powerless to break the patterns I had created myself.

I was a slave to email, social media messaging, and phone calls. Oh, and I'm not just talking on off-hours. My engagement continued around the clock and even on weekends.

Low-level anxiety became my way of life. It was the new normal for me. Anytime my cell phone beeped alerting me to a message, I couldn't resist the impulse to engage. I couldn't let messages go unanswered and I NEVER turned it off. This was partly because of my desire to please people and partly because answering my messages relieved my anxiety. My tech-addiction was flaring.

I used to blame others for messaging me at all hours of the day and night until I realized that it was my accessibility that gave them permission in the first place.

My awareness of this craziness prompted me to take action. I set boundaries and I began by respecting them myself. I set specific times for checking and responding. I let everyone in my life know my boundaries and now I don't blame anybody anymore for their expectations. Managing my life is my job and I am responsible for taking control. And so, I do. Although I still fight the temptation to engage.

I stopped thinking thoughts that brought on anxiety. I replaced them with new thoughts, reminding myself that I didn't need to be available to others 24/7. Today, I choose when I want to make myself available.

Instead of quelling my anxiety with my phone, I use essential oils to help calm me.

Do you have anxious feelings? Bergamot is a calming and uplifting oil. It can be soothing when you're feeling anxious or sad. Marjoram is valued for its calming properties and positive effect on the nervous system. Add to a soothing massage blend for targeting tired, stressed muscles. It may also promote healthy cardiovascular system function. Apply to the back of the neck to lessen feelings of stress.

Lavender and Wild Orange are also a couple of my go-tos, along with the blends I share in the book. It's important to remember that when it comes to maintaining a tranquil environment, it's all about balance.

Finding Balance

Have you ever felt like the world is crashing down on top of you? I have. If you're a mom, you have a major responsibility. In traditional families, there's the house and a family to care for, unless you can afford to hire help. How do you find balance?

If you have littles, there's school, and that comes with homework, doctor's appointments, play dates—you know the drill. And if you're a single parent, most of it falls on you. Balance? You're just trying to keep your head above water.

For moms who work jobs and momtrepreneurs, it can be especially challenging to find balance. We're last on the list, right? We have to keep things going at home while not missing a beat in our professional roles.

Believe me, I get it. Sometimes my life feels like a juggling act. If I were not laser-focused and committed, my life would probably fall apart. I would be living in complete pandemonium, unable to manage my time or my tasks.

Is balance important to me? I would say it's critical. I work to achieve it and maintain it. As I hinted in an earlier chapter, balance begins with organization.

If we're disorganized, our lives can be chaotic. Chaos can be super stressful, and that stress is there, bubbling under the surface, whether we're consciously aware of it or not.

Being unaware of how stressed we might be is more destructive than obvious forms of pressure because we inadvertently take it out on other people. Some stressors are out of our control, but being organized in the places we do have control can minimize the tension that sets us off. I'll give you an example.

Because I work from home, being organized means scheduling. It means list-making and having an orderly workspace. I want to know where everything is when I need it. Can I say this is super important because as a momtrepreneur, an organized workspace is the foundation I balance my life on. Order keeps me sane. If I'm stressed out and manic, that's not going to happen. Because guess what? Everything trickles down from the top; the good, the bad and the ugly. When my life is balanced, my family's lives are more balanced too.

And let me add this: it's not only about work. My home is also organized in such a way that things are comfortable and easy. I'm not obsessive compulsive, but I attribute much of my success to staying organized. My purse is always in the same place, and my cabinets are organized. The drawers in my bathroom are even organized.

And I cleanse by getting rid of anything I have not used in a few months. I can actually feel the difference energetically! Try it and see for yourself.

By the way, while you're de-cluttering your environment, grab a shovel and dig out of the mind-clutter you've been hoarding. I'll say it again. Wellness involves more than just a yearly physical, exercise and healthy eating. Mental and emotional stability are just as important. Clearing your mind is an important aspect of mental balance.

It's easy to allow overwhelm and responsibility to bury you. Make a commitment to yourself and clean your mental house every night before you go to bed.

And cut yourself some slack! Think about everything you have to do in a single day. If you listed every task you complete from the time you get out of bed until you turn off the lights at night, you'd probably be stunned by how much you actually do. How the heck DO you manage to get all of it done? Well, sometimes you get things done and sometimes you don't. If you do a daily clearing, you'll avoid having those "don'ts" add up and stare you in the face the next day. You'll bring yourself back into what? Right! Balance.

Our thoughts are central to maintaining balance. Get in the habit of monitoring your thoughts. That's where change begins. You need to know where you are before you determine where you want to go next. Your thoughts will take you there.

Melissa essential oil is good for support. Add Melissa to a moisturizer or a spray bottle with water and spritz on your face to rejuvenate skin and refresh your thoughts.

Melissa calms tension and nerves and promotes relaxation. Diffuse Melissa at night or rub it on your forehead, shoulders, or chest to lessen stress and promote emotional well-being. Diffuse it anytime to uplift your mood.

Harboring Resentment

Do you harbor resentment when you get angry? I hope not. Resentment is toxic! It feels horrible. Instead of letting go of emotional pain, resentment causes you to replay feelings of anger or memories of events that brought those muddy feelings about in the first place. So not good for you!

Essential oils will assist you in the process of releasing the toxic emotions that darken your life. Look through the section on essential oils blends or use oils with calming properties. I use a special renewing blend for forgiveness. It helps to counteract emotions of anger and guilt, while promoting the liberating feelings of contentment, relief, and patience. Love it, love it.

Do you like the scent of Patchouli? It has a musky-sweet aroma. Older hippies will remember it from the 70s. When things are rocky, add three to four drops in a diffuser to help ground and balance your emotions. I LOVE adding a drop of Wild Orange and even Lime to Patchouli to sweeten it up a bit. My days with The Grateful Dead are over, LOL. I need a slightly different angle on the aroma of Patchouli straight up.

A bonus is that Patchouli promotes a smooth, glowing complexion. You've gotta love those double benefits!

I have question for you. Are you angry with yourself over something you've done? Have you made a mistake and you're having trouble forgiving yourself? That's resentment.

You know, everybody slips up once in a while.

Subconsciously, resentment can cause you to judge yourself harshly and self-judgment is unhealthy. It's often the source of feelings of undeserving. When you feel unworthy, you might self-sabotage when good things come your way. Meditation is helpful in bringing you back to center. Diffuse Sandalwood and maybe Frankincense while you meditate. They are frequently used in meditation for their grounding properties.

Regardless of what you've done, forgive yourself and let go. Start over with new, productive thoughts.

Here's what can happen if you don't choose your thoughts consciously....

What Are You Thinking?

Have you ever tried to consciously examine your thoughts? You know, think about what you're thinking? What are you saying to yourself?

These are important questions because your thoughts dictate your reality. Are you telling yourself you can have and do anything you choose, or the opposite? I'll promise you this: if you're telling yourself you will never have what you want, chances are you won't.

If you believe you don't deserve good things for whatever reason, you'll push away every opportunity that could move you closer to your dream come true. Your thoughts reflect everything you believe about yourself. So, if your thoughts aren't getting you what you want, it might be time to change them.

Pay attention to what you think—about life, about people, about money—and then change the thoughts that hold you back. Yep, it's that simple. Pick a new thought to believe instead of an old story you've been telling yourself for who knows how long. And see, the thing is, what we are thinking then has an impact on our emotions or how we feel.

So this is where essential oils come in and make it all a bit easier for you. You see, the sense of smell exerts control over our emotions. It connects us with our memories and thoughts. Certain aromatherapy blends can elevate mood and enhance emotional well-being. So yes, try to live your life being more "conscious"—literally. But in addition, try allowing the aromatherapy to give you a boost.

It doesn't matter where you are in life. You're not stuck. You're one single second away from shift and change in any direction. Be conscious of your starting point and decide which way you want to go.

Always pay attention to what's going on between your ears. Add Thyme to favorite daytime diffuser blends to promote a sense of alertness. Be aware of where your mind takes you and think your way to the life you want to experience.

CHAPTER FOUR

Seeing is Believing... or is Believing, Seeing?

THE PROVERB, *Seeing is Believing*, refers to the concept that you need to see something before you can accept that it really exists. You know, like the old *Doubting Thomas* adage. The place to start is to examine the thoughts you have and then work directly with your belief system. I call this "consciously waking up."

It goes both ways; believing is also seeing. When you believe you will have, do, or be anything, you will have the power to make it a reality. Regardless of what anyone has told you, you really are in control.

Mind if I segue a minute? I'm going to get technical for a sec, but I promise what I have to tell you is a valuable part of your essential oils journey and I would be remiss not to include it here. I'm sure you'll find this info super interesting, too.

This section has a lot to do with understanding ways essential oils can benefit your life, and so I don't want to gloss over it. When I decided to write this book, I wanted to be sure to clue you in on more than simply how to use essential oils or where to apply them. I want you to understand the benefits of oils so you'll get the full value of your experience. Oils can be a big part of major life change as I pointed out with my personal story. Your story is just as important.

Essential oils do more than smell good (or in some cases, not so good). Along with your thoughts, they impact your life experience in four realms: mental, physical, emotional, and spiritual. Thoughts dictate your actions and your actions define you. Everything works together.

Where Do Thoughts Come From?

Have you ever stopped to think about where your thoughts come from? They don't just pop into your head out of nowhere. Or do they?

Thoughts are things. Positive thoughts can create positive change and negative thoughts can have serious effects on your health and well-being. But the process doesn't stop with you. Your states of being, positive and negative, affect the people around you. So, it's a big deal.

You believe what you tell yourself by affirming your thoughts with self-talk. That's the voice inside your head. As long as you spew positivity, or even neutrality, you're in good shape. Positive self-talk generates positive results. But negative self-talk is a vehicle of self-sabotage.

I'd like to point out that I don't believe people have to walk around thinking only positive thoughts. Like I said a minute ago, our thoughts are sometimes neutral.

For instance, if I'm flying on an airline and I ordered a vegetarian meal and it didn't appear on my flight, I can choose the thought, "this airline is incompetent" or I can choose the thought "the agent may not have heard me when I requested my meal." It's not necessarily a positive thought. It's just a new thought that will prevent me from getting upset with the airline, right?

If you allow negative thoughts to stick around, they can lead to physical ailments such as headaches, digestive issues, and insomnia. Allergies and panic attacks are also associated with negative thought patterns. In worst-case scenarios, obsessing with negativity can lead to panic attacks and even heart problems.

Negativity is toxic. Using essential oils can support wellness practices and aid in detoxifying. But why not also head disease off at the pass by training yourself to think good thoughts from the beginning?

How can you do this? The answer is simple, but it's not necessarily easy to lock in as a habit. It takes practice. The place to start is to examine the thoughts you have and then work directly with your belief system.

Your beliefs are assumptions you make about life. They are not always true, even though you may THINK they are. They are values you hold about yourself, others, and the world around you.

Wait! Some of your beliefs are totally of base. Yet they are constantly affecting your life whether you are aware of them or not. Read on. I'll explain what I mean.

Some beliefs develop early in life and are reinforced through experiences and situations you confront throughout your life. They are strongly held and inflexible unless you examine them and work to change them. If you try something new and fail, you might tell yourself "I can't do that," even before you try. You believe your assumption. See how dangerous this type of thinking can be?

If you hold a belief that you're unlikable, no matter how many people tell you otherwise, you won't own it because your thoughts are that you are unlikable. You discount compliments, feel embarrassed or distrust people who say they like you. You'll do whatever it takes to prove your belief that you are unlikable right.

Not all beliefs are negative. You hold beliefs about positive aspects of yourself and life, too. It goes both ways. They can help you create success or they can be on the front line as you sabotage your good fortune. If one of your beliefs is that money is dirty, or that you are unworthy of wealth, no matter how much good you attract, you'll push it away every time just so you can prove your belief about money true. At the same time, if you believe money comes easily to you, it will. If you believe you are strong; resilient; you will be. You will think thoughts that reinforce those beliefs.

Are you still with me? It's super important that you understand this concept because your belief system is the guiding force in your life. It's where (some of) your thoughts come from. Your thoughts support your beliefs. Now, it would be great if all your thoughts were true. As I said, they're not.

Some thoughts can be life changing. Others push you so far off course that even a ton of work and a firm essential oils regimen won't get back to where you need to be. Can thoughts be that powerful? Yes! Let's explore why.

What Exactly Are Thoughts?

Thoughts aren't tangible. They are abstract states of mind. They respond to stimuli from your personal experience and from bits of information placed into your belief system by others. Your thoughts are connected to everything you're associated with—your environment, your impressions and your perceptions.

Some thoughts are fleeting wisps of information. These are neutral thoughts.

> "There's a tree!"
> "I'm cold."
> "The sky is blue."

Thoughts determine your results. Not happy with your life? Change your thoughts. Seriously, how do you do that? By changing your beliefs!

If your thoughts just floated around in your head, it would be bad enough. But they don't. What you THINK often comes spilling out of your mouth. Your thoughts become your words.

Your THOUGHTS create your actions and your actions lead to results. They determine the way you relate to others. You can motivate yourself to do things—even things you never thought you could do—by changing your thoughts.

Your words impact your emotions and how you feel about yourself. They can also influence how those around you think and feel. Words are indicators of what's going on inside your head. You share your feelings with words.

How do you feel about yourself? What do you think about others? Your thoughts and words answer these questions.

Watch what you think.
Pay attention to the words that come from your thoughts.
Be aware of the actions that follow your words.

Okay, now let's look at how you can support your positive life change with essential oils.

Which Essential Oils Support Positive Thinking?

Making changes in your life, even on as basic a level as your thoughts, requires assertiveness. You'll need to make decisions and then be strong as you make those changes. Basil is an essential oil that encourages assertiveness. If you get easily confused and have a tough time making decisions, it's a good one to work with.

Making deep and profound changes sometimes disrupts a family system. If no one else in your family or circle is working on the same type of change, you might not get a lot of support from those closest to you. Essential oils will aid you in hanging tough when you need to. Diffuse Fennel with Basil. This blend helps ward off negative thoughts of others and keep you from absorbing other people's toxicity.

Do you like black licorice? Then you'll love fennel. Blend fennel with fractionated coconut oil for a soothing massage. Diffuse Fennel in your home or office to encourage a productive day.

Basil has a warm and spicy, yet herbal aroma. It acts as a cooling agent for the skin. Basil promotes mental alertness and lessens occasional anxious feelings. Diffuse it to promote a sense of focus while studying, reading, or completing other tasks that require mental clarity. Massage Basil and Wintergreen with Fractionated Coconut Oil on the back of the neck for a stress-relieving experience.

Can Oils Offer Emotional and Spiritual Support?

The answer is yes. Absolutely. Here are some of my favorites.

I love Frankincense! It elevates the spirit and promotes clarity of mind. Use it to reinforce your efforts toward personal and spiritual growth. Blend with sandalwood, which helps to increase feelings of peace and tranquility. This is a super combo to diffuse during meditation.

Change comes with a few challenges. Even making positive changes can bring on feelings of sadness as you let go of the familiar. Roman Chamomile has a soothing effect on both mind and body. Put a few drops behind your ears to increase feelings of inner peace, serenity and emotional stability.

It goes without saying that change can be stressful. Are you going through a rough time and feeling emotionally exhausted? Sad? Even positive change can ripple out to affect other areas of your life and result in tension.

Bergamot and Roman Chamomile are wonderful oils. Keep them in stock, along with Geranium, which aids in dissolving frustration and helps you stay centered.

Don't let stress get the best of you! Here's an idea. Try blending Geranium with Bergamot and relaxing in a hot bath. Use them together in a diffuser. They smell yummy and both offer powerful support for bringing you back into balance.

Now, you'll read a lot about Lavender in my book so don't be surprised. That's because it is such a versatile oil. If I could suggest only one oil, (which would never happen), I would say Lavender is a must-have oil. It has several applications, and the most critical in this context would be that it helps clear away negative thoughts. It also aids in dispelling worry and apprehension.

Does a troubled mind keep you awake at night? Lavender is again, unparalleled. Diffuse it in your bedroom or spray it on your pillow. I know people who do this, and they say the moment they lay their heads down they are sound asleep. If you wake up a lot during the night and your mind movies start running, a sniff of Lavender will calm you and help you get back to sleep.

Life Happens

No matter what you do to stay centered and balanced, life is going to happen around you. Some things are mind-blowing amazing, and others can be devastating. How do you respond when life collapses on top of you?

A wellness regimen will definitely make a difference when you're brought face-to-face with distress, but some things shake you so hard they can wipe away all that positive thinking and thrust you back into survival mode. It doesn't matter what's happening; your *perception* of what's going on takes over. You process the situation and then thoughts direct your actions as you respond—or react—to what you believe to be true.

When we're in survival mode, we often revert to what we are most comfortable with. That's usually what we know best. We think and act on autopilot until we bring ourselves back into balance. Essential oils to the rescue!

Do you drink tea? Change regular tea to Earl Grey tea with the addition of Bergamot. Apply Bergamot to your feet before bedtime for a sense of calm and harmony. Bergamot mixes well with Lavender, Patchouli, Lime, Arborvitae, Ylang Ylang, and Frankincense.

Addiction

You might discover you're addicted to a particular thought pattern because somewhere along the line there's a payoff. The payoff might be in the form of validation of a core value. If you believe you are not smart, you might become addicted to thoughts that reinforce the belief by prompting results that prove it. Even negative, self-sabotaging beliefs can be magnetic if they serve a purpose.

As you explore your thoughts and beliefs, if you discover any kind of attachment, and you want to make a change,

Cypress is the oil for you. You might be feeling vulnerable and insecure about walking a new road and this oil offers a feeling of protection. It helps you achieve balance and inner peace as well as confidence when making changes. Blend it with Ylang Ylang; it is also good for boosting self-confidence. And if you know anyone working to break an addiction, Cypress is the perfect gift.

There's A Way Out

Are you done struggling? You'll know it when you are. You're never stuck with a belief system that no longer fits, or thoughts that keep you down. If you're ready to move forward to the life waiting for you, it's time to clean out the closet and rid yourself of any thought, belief or habit that holds you back from having what you desire and deserve.

Where do you begin?

Get to know yourself. The better you understand the person you are and your thoughts the easier it will be to change. Peppermint is a good companion oil for this type of self-discovery. It increases sensitivity and awareness. And grab that bottle of Bergamot again. Diffuse it for a sense of self-confidence as you make your changes.

I am committed to positive thinking, and so I start my day with Frankincense, Wild Orange and Bergamot. Mix Frankincense with anything and the properties are enhanced. Check out the blends in the last chapter for a few more ideas.

Chapter Five

Essential Oils Can Help You Cope With Stress and Anxious Feelings

THE WORD *stress* has become a part of every day language. People at increasingly younger ages are getting zapped by it and its effects are far reaching. Everyday experiences, work responsibilities and serious life events all trigger stress.

What is Stress?

Stress is more than a nervous condition resulting in emotional discomfort. If you ignore it for very long symptoms can result in serious health issues. Symptoms of stress include—but are not limited to—upset stomach, headache, and fatigue. When you're stressed, you may notice a change in appetite or high levels of anxious feelings.

Stress and anxiety though related, are not the same. The difference between stress and anxiety is that stress is a response to a perceived threat and anxiety is a reaction to the stress. For example, if you are afraid of spiders, it might be *stressful* to walk in the woods, especially if you see one or two along the way. You might become *anxious* if you spot a spider web as you continue your walk.

I don't know anyone who can say they live a completely stress-free life. I would say some people can handle their stress better than others, but nobody I know sails through life without a little drama now and then.

These are busy, complicated times and it can be hard to maintain balance. Your best defense is to minimize stress by assuming control of your life. This begins with, what else? Your thoughts! No matter how well controlled you are, challenging circumstances will squeeze through the cracks of your life. Stress is inevitable. Learning how to harness the healing power of essential oils will help you cope.

Here are a few tips that when combined with an essential oils regimen will help you manage stress.

Manage Your Perceptions

What's your outlook on life? You might see it as a wild adventure, or serious and lesson-packed. Whatever it is, your point of view will dictate how you interpret your experience of life. An interpretation is not necessarily fact. Remember, things are not always as we think they are. Much of what we perceive to be true is based upon assumptions or fantasy. Even when they're not real, those made-up stories can cause stress.

Certain medical conditions associated with stress can wear you down and others can be debilitating. Irritable Bowel Discomfort or autoimmunity, both rooted in stress, can making it difficult or impossible to live a normal life.

Other conditions can be deadly. Stress has been linked to heart attacks and it may also prompt a stroke or cancer. Any way you look at it, no amount of stress is good.

Essential oils have long been used for calming and relaxation; by themselves or in conjunction with other wellness strategies. Here are a few of the most popular and effective approaches.

Ahhh...Massage

No doubt about it, even a simple back rub or neck massage feels great. When you work with a skilled masseur or masseuse, even better. Massage is relaxing and rejuvenating, and one of my favorite go-tos when I am feeling stressed—and even when I'm not.

Among other things, massage can help to:

Ease Muscle Pain
Alleviate Tension
Reduce Headache Pain
Relieve Back and Neck Pain
Strengthen the Immune System
Improve Nerve Function

The History of Massage

I don't know a lot about massage, other than I LOVE it, but here's a little background.

Massage has its roots in both eastern and western culture. I can imagine people were doing massage long before they learned how to write, but the benefits of massage have been documented for over 4,000 years. Today's research continues proves that this ancient practice really does help nurture and maintain wellness.

Massage helps reduce stress and tension, the number one causes of disease. It also strengthens the immune system and energizes the mind. You know the old saying, "a flexible body means a flexible mind."

It's super important to drink fluids after a massage so your body can eliminate lactic acid and toxins released by the massage. There are several types of massage used for different issues.

Swedish Massage

A popular method of massage used for relaxation or following exercise is Swedish massage. This gentle, soothing touch relaxes aching muscles and relieves tension. It has also been known to increase range of motion and many chiropractors even offer it to patients in their offices following treatment.

Swedish massage is effective for pain relief. When combined with clinical trigger point therapy (in the shoulders, hip and lower back), pain can be reduced or eliminated altogether.

Therapeutic Massage

Massage is so much more than a feel-good experience. It can also be therapeutic by helping improve and maintain a healthy body, mind and spirit. Therapeutic massage helps to create a sense of physical, mental and emotional well-being. When combined with essential oils, the benefits can be magnified. In fact, some massage therapists use aromatherapy by diffusing essential oils in their treatment rooms.

Massage for Insomnia

Do you toss and turn at night? Find it hard to fall asleep? Well, stress can keep you up at night. Even if you're able to fall asleep, stress can wake you up after a couple hours and then keep you from falling back to sleep. You toss and turn and then the thoughts start: about what you have to do the next day, what's wrong with your life, or any problems you're facing. Massage is useful because it helps to facilitate better sleep patterns. Lavender essential oil blended with a base oil is an awesome combination with a back rub before bed.

Lymphatic Massage

Your lymphatic system helps eliminate waste. By improving circulation of lymphatic fluid, massage helps your body fight off infection. Some doctors suggest a specific process called lymphatic drainage massage after surgery.

So, we all agree that massage is a benefit, right? There's only one problem: professional massage can be expensive and depending on your budget you may or may not be able to afford weekly or even monthly massage. In that case, trading shoulder rubs with a friend can be helpful for both of you. Of course, adding essential oils makes it even better.

Blend these oils in your next massage: Spruce, Frankincense, Blue Tansy, Blue Chamomile, and Fractionated Coconut oil. A popular blend for massage also incorporates the relaxing properties of Cypress plant, Peppermint plant, Marjoram leaf, Basil leaf, Grapefruit peel, and Lavender flower essential oils.

Take up Yoga

Okay, so now we're on my turf again. Yoga is one of my passions—I taught Yoga and Pilates for fifteen years and still practice every day. If you're already dabbling in Yoga, you know how useful it is for stress reduction. And if you've never done it or you're just getting started, I have good news! You don't have to work up to the benefits of Yoga. Even beginners feel the benefits immediately.

Any type of exercise is essential to health and wellness, can we agree on that? We're talking balance here. Yoga is a popular form of exercise—and meditation—based on centuries-old eastern traditions. But it's not just a physical activity. It will help you balance your life because it's a body-mind-spirit practice.

How did Yoga work its way westward?

East met west (and Yoga) through American-born Richard Hittleman, who studied Yoga in India. He promoted Hatha Yoga in the United States during the 50s–70s. Although it's not the only style of Yoga practiced in the United States, Hatha Yoga is the best-known form of Yoga in western culture. Other Yoga styles, such as Ashtanga (vigorous) and relaxing Restorative styles, are super popular. All Yoga styles emphasize sustained poses and specialized breathing techniques.

What are the benefits of stretches, poses, and bends such as the Butterfly and the Crane? What about Yoga's focused breathing techniques? How do they help with stress?

Well, Yoga can't stop someone from getting on your nerves. That's the job of your thoughts. But it can reduce feelings of stress through mindful relaxation techniques. The increased strength and improved flexibility from Yoga can also help your body cope with and recover from daily stress.

Almost everyone knows the standard advice about starting a new exercise program and you've probably heard it, too. Check with your doctor, wear appropriate clothing and stay hydrated.

Don't just jump into a class without doing a little digging. It's important to know the style and philosophy of your Yoga instructor before starting a class. You're more likely to keep doing something if you like it.

Hot Yoga classes are really getting popular. It's *literally* hot. Rooms hosting Hot Yoga are typically heated to increase sweating. You might prefer a Yoga routine with a focus on physical exercise rather than mediation. Checking with the instructor or buds who have already taken a specific instructor's class can help you strike the right pose for you.

Oh, and buy your own mat. It's more sanitary. If you have to share, clean it well between users.

Stress-Reducing Essential Oils

There are tons of brands of essential oils on the market and they run the gamut between cheap-and-cheesy and high quality. You can buy them online and in stores. Be sure to learn about oils before you choose a brand. The certified pure theraputic grade (CPTG) oils are best. But remember to use all oils with care. Even essential oils can be harmful if you don't use them properly.

Using essential oils for stress management can involve everything from sniffing, rolling on, bathing, diffusing and other methods. Go ahead and use them in cooking. I've included recipes so read on. Put a few drops your faves in your morning coffee or tea. You might even enjoy them in your oatmeal—try Wild Orange, Peppermint, or Bergamot.

Making essential oils a part of your life will definitely change your health for the better and your stress levels will go way down. It doesn't matter if you are young or old. Oils are used to help kids focus and Lavender is specifically used to soothe crying babies. Lavender scented baby lotion is awesome.

Is this all woo-woo crazy stuff? Absolutely not. There's scientific proof. Essential oil therapy, also called aromatherapy has been found to alter brain waves and behavior. It can reduce the perception of stress, which means it has an effect on the way you interpret what's going on around you.

Keep this top of mind: stress, especially prolonged stress, can be harmful. It really doesn't matter what method you choose to manage it. Just do something. Minimize stress before it takes over, but if you're already dealing with it, this chapter has a lot of good ideas to help you manage. Even if you do nothing else, using essential oils by themselves is hugely beneficial.

Chapter Six

How Essential Oils Can Help Relieve Anxious Feelings and Sadness

NOW, WE all experience anxious feelings and sadness, right? When we're concerned about a situation we're going through or nervous about an upcoming event, anxious feelings are common. Physiologically, anxious feelings are usually caused by the release of adrenaline in response to fear.

If we are unhappy, we feel sad. Now, sadness is appropriate in some cases and not necessarily bad unless it overwhelms us or prevents us from living fully. All of our emotions have a purpose. It's only when they're out of whack that they become detrimental.

Although essential oils can help provide symptom relief for both anxious or sad feelings, it can also be helpful to talk with a friend or someone you trust when you're feeling blue.

More than ever before, anxiety and depression are at the forefront of discussions in the professional and private sectors. Even though the two are characterized by different symptoms, if you suffer from one there is often evidence of the other.

Anxiety can be debilitating, especially if worry gnaws at you. Fear, whether real or imagined, is overwhelming and can rob you of happiness. That's why anxious feelings often lead to sadness.

If your sadness is persistent it can result in appetite changes, fatigue, sleep difficulties, low self-esteem, feelings of hopelessness and poor concentration.

Again, if you are experiencing any of the symptoms above, ask for support from someone you trust. Once you have that worked out, essential oil remedies can help with symptom relief. There's even been some research on this.

Studies have shown an essential oil blend of Bergamot, Frankincense and Lavender to support a healthy mood. Diffuse it if you like, or massage the blend into your hands or bottoms of your feet.

I'm sure I don't have to tell you, waking up to today's world is nothing like a day at Disneyland. All you have to do is read the paper or watch the news and you'll easily understand why so many people are suffering.

I'm not just referencing the state of affairs around the planet, or, depending on where in the world you live, even your own country. I'm not even talking about what's happening in your neighborhood, around the block, or right next door. I'm referring to what's going on behind your own front door.

We all have tension in our personal lives. Whether we are worrying about paying bills and making monthly rent or mortgage payments, or whether we're concerned about what's going on with family members or friends dealing with their own issues. What happens to those anxious feelings? Unless we deal with them, they can make us miserable, right?

So where do you turn? I mean, these feelings are not going away on their own. If you don't face your feelings head on, they will grab you by your vulnerability, take hold and shake; or you'll repress them, and they will make you sick.

One of the ways I deal with my upsets is through prayer and meditation. What if you're not religious? It doesn't matter. Even if you don't believe in God, pray to a higher power. No matter what your religious affiliation, prayer and meditation can help dissolve sadness or anger or any other negative emotion. They are spiritual tools.

Dealing with pressure is a lot easier if you can get outside yourself—or, more accurately, *inside* yourself. Meditation is a super effective way to calm your nerves and put you in touch with the power of your unconscious mind. It can relieve that vexing tension and free you to handle the challenges that end up on your doorstep. Diffuse your favorite oils during meditation. Try Rose, Jasmine and other floral oils.

Learning to meditate is not complicated. It's super simple. If you keep up with it, you can refine over time. You can pray or meditate any time, anywhere. Meditate while you hike, or on a run.

If you prefer, you can meditate in a more formal setting. Find a comfortable place to sit, recline or lie down. It's helpful to create a sacred space to use only when you meditate. The benefit? You'll find yourself beginning to relax even before you start your meditation. Your body/mind system will remember subconsciously and respond. The same goes for the oils you use during your quiet time. I often use Frankincense, Myrrh or Sandalwood.

In your space, surround yourself with favorite objects and things that make you feel peaceful. Play soft mood music if you like. This is your little corner of the world; a place where you are in control. Create your own space and your own experience.

When you're ready to begin your meditation, get comfortable and close your eyes. Take a few cleansing breaths. Listen to a guided meditation or sit in silence. Meditation is generally an emptying of the mind. It can also be a kind of self-guided imagery, or self-hypnosis and can involve a progressive relaxation if you like. That's a process of relaxing your body a section at a time. Again, your choice.

Because body, mind, and spirit are all connected, prayer and meditation can provide huge benefits. They help to lower your oxygen consumption, decrease your respiratory rate, and increase blood flow.

Sometimes five or ten minutes off the grid focusing inward can take you to another plane. If you practice meditation regularly, you'll soon find that you feel less anxious and more relaxed. You'll be more able to cope with the challenges that come your way.

Isolating yourself when you feel low can make your world a very small place. It can crush your resolve and your determination to have what you want. You deserve to live a full, beautiful life. Do everything you can to grab hold and then bring your dreams into reality.

NOTE: Do not rely on essential oils to cure or heal you if you experience anxiety or depression. Seek professional help. Once you are getting the support you need for anxiety and depression, essential oil remedies can help with symptom relief.

Chapter Seven

Releasing Negative Emotions

DO YOU like being around negative people? Never mind. I already know the answer. None of us do. It's worse if you're the one being negative.

A negative disposition only makes you and others around you miserable—that is if people are still around you. If people see you as negative they may run for the hills when they see you coming. Negativity can result in a very lonely life. You may not even like being around you, but you're stuck unless you change your thoughts.

Holding on to negativity takes up a ton of emotional space. But there's hope if you're willing to release it. By releasing negative emotions such as bitterness, anger and resentment you will make space in your head and in your heart. You'll be able to love more. You'll have less stress and when something heavy does come along, you'll have the resources to deal with it. Anger can lead to resentment if not dealt with and both point directly to bitterness.

What is Anger?

Is anger bad? As children a lot of us are taught that anger is not polite. Hold it in. Swallow it. Don't express it. Right; like it goes away when we do that. All these lead to is passive aggression or turning that anger inward against ourselves. And then so many of us spend the majority of our adult lives learning how to identify and feel our feelings and then express them appropriately.

The truth is, anger in and of itself is not necessarily a negative emotion. It has a purpose. Anger a strong feeling we have in response to something that upsets us. *Upset* can range in intensity from slight irritation to powerful rage, with many feelings in between. Here's an example.

When you lock your keys in your car you might feel irritated. If you have another set in your purse or brief case, you might be inconvenienced but also relieved, so your upset is minimal and diffuses easily. Now if you own only one set of keys, and the only way to retrieve it is to call AAA or another service for help and then wait for them to get to you, you'd be a little more upset; maybe aggravated.

Let's up the game.

Add the fact that you will be late for a job interview, or that it's after midnight. Now you might be exasperated or seriously pissed off about the situation. If you've also locked your cell phone in the car and the door to the building you've just exited locked behind you, and you might be enraged. Each of these emotions is on the spectrum of anger. This is why what you tell yourself is important:

Who cares if you're keys are locked in the car? Or that you left your phone in there too? Or that you're late for a job interview? Well, YOU do obviously, because of what you're choosing to believe:

I can't get into my car without my keys.

I need to get in my car to go home or to the interview. I will never get out of here without my car or being able to call someone to rescue me.

There is no way I'll get this job interview unless I get into my car right now.

If I don't get the job my life is going to end.

My point is, if you're thoughts were:

I really have nowhere to go.

I actually wanted to explore this town anyway. I'll mosey down the street and eventually find a phone and ask someone to pick me up.

I didn't really want to go to that interview anyway. In fact, I don't really want to get ANY job. I love the freedom in my life.

This is such a fantastic opportunity to be completely off the grid for a few hours!

...then there would be no anger, right?

One face of anger comes with major ramifications, and that's rage. Again, the expression of anger, apart from rage, can actually be super healthy. It may even help you think more rationally. But if you allow anger to simmer, and if you hold it in or explode in rage, you can make yourself really sick. Really, really sick.

What do I mean by this? Worst-case scenario, rage or angry outbursts can put you at risk of heart attack. In fact, it doubles your chances. Repressed anger is anger you either express indirectly, such as being passive aggressive, or anger you bury. Either one doubles your risk of coronary disease or stroke.

If you also have other health symptoms that increase the odds, you could be putting your life in danger. I'd say that's pretty serious, wouldn't you?

How can you protect yourself? You can't stop from having feelings, even angry feelings. Emotions are responses. If you don't allow them, you might repress them. What you can do is learn to recognize your feelings before they swell into rage. If you notice that you're feeling angry about something, acknowledge it and then deal with it appropriately. What are you thinking about the situation? Can you replace it with another thought?

We all know people who go through life just plain angry. They wake up mad and go to bed mad. They're upset when you say no, and they're upset when you say yes. You can't win because they will be angry no matter what. People who live angry lives are not doing themselves any favor. I'll tell you why.

Anger might be justified in some cases, but it doesn't mean you need to hold onto it forever. You only harm yourself. Your immune system will be lower, and so you might find yourself getting sick more often. A Harvard University study once found that even when people were not necessarily angry, but recalled an episode that upset them, their levels of antibodies that fight disease went down for several hours. And they weren't even angry to begin with! A friggin' memory caused the reaction.

Letting Go of Anger

Learning how to cope with your emotions will help you deal with anger appropriately. One of those ways is to maintain a balanced lifestyle. Of course—ta-da—essential oils are part of that prescription! There are a few super awesome essential oils to keep on hand, not just in case of emergency, but for every day use.

Anger raises your blood pressure and heart rate and so when I am upset, or my kids are freaking out over something, remember my go-to when I need calming? Yep. Lavender and Wild Orange to the rescue!

Under a lot of stress? Add Ylang Ylang to the mix. It will help lessen tension and relieve stress. If you're feeling down because of a situation you're angry about, Ylang Ylang will help elevate your mood.

Something to keep in mind: anger is a secondary emotion masking fear and/or sadness. When you feel angry about something, ask yourself if you might be feeling sad or scared or a little of both. If so try an elevating blend containing Lavender Flower, Hawaiian Sandalwood, Tangerine Peel, Melissa Flower, Ylang Ylang Flower, Elemi Resin, Osmanthus Flower, and Lemon Myrtle Leaf essential oils. It will help bring you back into balance by elevating your mood and relieving anxious feelings.

Something you probably already know about anger is it makes you want to munch. There's a reason for that. Well, actually, there are a couple reasons. Chewing crunchy things or biting a lot helps relief pressure. Eating also helps you swallow those feelings you really need to be expressing. Along with your essential oils regime, be sure you eat a diet low in processed sugar. Crunch an apple, not chips.

Remember anger is natural. It's a part of the fight-flight response in times we feel threatened. If you are lacking in vitamins and minerals you can feel high levels of anxiety that keep you in a constant state of unease and poised for confrontation—even when there's nothing to be angry about. Make sure you take supplements and eat healthy foods. Add your essential oils to fresh vegetable salads for another way to consume them and for unique flavor enhancements.

Zinc is another good choice especially for women. (But go ahead, guys. It can't hurt.) Studies with both women and female animals show that zinc helps with feelings of anger and anxiety.

B vitamins have several health benefits. They can also help you deal with repressed anger. B vitamins include thiamine, riboflavin, niacin or niacinamide. They also include vitamin B6, vitamin B12, folic acid, and pantothenic acid. B-complex helps by lowering homocysteine levels. What does that mean?

Although results are still seen as inconclusive, high levels of homocysteine may lead to heart disease. Strokes, osteoporosis, Crohn's disease, Alzheimer's disease, diabetes, miscarriages, and hypothyroidism are also indirectly risks of holding onto repressed anger. Vitamin B-complex is a known remedy for lowering homocysteine levels.

Is All Anger a Threat to Good Health?

Not all types of anger do harm. Constructive anger is not associated with heart disease. Why not? Because it's productive. When you are upset by something another person has said or done, talk to the person you're upset with. Face your feelings head on instead of burying them. Let the person know how you feel about what they may have done or said. Do this for you, not for them. You can't control the reactions of another. Express and release.

And while we're talking about this, remember people don't *make you feel* anything. You make you feel. Take responsibility for your feelings. Don't blame or guilt-trip others. That comes from either a victim mentality or it's passive aggressive. Relieve yourself of anger before it becomes resentment.

Resentment is super toxic. It's the process of repetitively replaying the feelings of anger or the events that brought them about in the first place. By doing so we force ourselves to relive the experience emotionally, mentally—and even physically.

Regardless of whether we are hurt or angry, allowing the actions of another to occupy our hearts and minds only hurts us. The only way out is to release. It may seem as though you're doing it for the other person, but you're actually doing it for yourself.

Release Negativity Through Forgiveness

Just in case you think the word *forgive* means "letting the other guy off the hook," or "sweep it under the carpet," it doesn't. Now, it could mean, "bury the hatchet," but not in the other person's back!

Forgive actually translates as "to free." The Greek translation means "to let go." Letting go of negativity frees emotional space and can have HUGE health benefits as well. It's an essential part of wellness.

Where do you start? Well, why not begin by forgiving yourself?

Huh?

Yep. Whether we're aware of it or not, we all hold on to resentment against ourselves: for mistakes we've made or bad behaviors. We resent the times we've said things we shouldn't have or stayed in relationships we knew were bad for us. These resentments cause us to judge ourselves, and judgment calls for punishment. This is often the source of feelings of undeserving and self-sabotage.

Let Go!

I use an awesome blend from the company I purchase my oils from and have chosen to partner with. It helps counteract emotions of anger and guilt. (By the way guilt is anger turned inward.) Ingredients are: Spruce Leaf, Bergamot Peel, Juniper Berry Fruit, Myrrh Resin, Arborvitae Wood, Nootka Tree Wood, Thyme Leaf, Citronella Herb.

Regardless of what you've done or said in the past, it's behind you now. Forgive and forget. Don't relive the past in your mind. Save that place for your dreams.

Chapter Eight

Essential Oils for Health and Wellness

OUR ANCESTORS turned to essential oils for so many reasons, including the soothing and purifying qualities they have on the skin, and also of course, their calming effect. But as you're going to see in this chapter, there are plenty of other unique ways to use oils for overall wellness.

There are a variety of ways to use these products, but use them with caution if you have skin sensitivity. One of the benefits of essential oils is their versatility. Whether you have dry skin, oily skin, or skin that's irritated, there is an essential oil you can use to soothe, moisturize and cleanse your face or other parts of your body.

If you have littles running around the house, remember they like to explore. Most essential oils smell like they also probably taste good, and kids can be drawn to them for that reason. Please keep them out of the reach of children. Also, even though pure oils (CPTG) are generally safe for topical use, some are full-strength, and the rule doesn't hold. Avoid getting them in your eyes, inner ears, or other sensitive areas. And needless to say, if you are pregnant or under a doctor's care, consult your physician before using essential oils.

As a beginner with essential oils, there is also a lot to learn. Once you get some practice, it will be smooth sailing from there. As you get started, it's important for you to know about certain essential oils you can use as part of your overall wellness regime. So, I put this list together for you. Check it out. You might also see a few of these oils on other lists. That's because of their versatility. You'll also notice there are several oils you can use to relieve tension.

BASIL

This is a good place to start. As you've figured out by now after reading the last couple chapters, we all deal with stress, and depending on our lifestyles, some of us more than others. Basil is a good oil to keep on hand.

Basil offers a warm and spicy aroma that will definitely produce a calming effect and can reduce stress levels. Its high linalool content makes it ideal for reducing feelings of tension when applied to the temples and back of the neck. You can also combine it with Geranium and Wild Orange essential oils. It makes for the perfect aromatic massage! And as you'll learn, Basil oil is tasty when you use it in Italian cooking.

BERGAMOT

So, this is one of the more unique citrus oils. Bergamot can be both calming and uplifting at the same time. That's why this is a great oil for balance. Earl Grey must have realized that when he put it in his tea. Bergamot is perfect for those days when you're feeling sad or having anxious feelings.

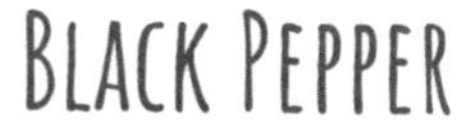

Black Pepper

All these years you've been peppering your food and I'll bet you didn't know you were also aiding digestion. This essential oil promotes healthy circulation and can also aid with the digestion of foods. All in all, it's a perfect oil to cook with. You'll be getting great flavor and healthy internal benefits at the same time!

Cardamom

This oil has a lot of health benefits that many don't know about. Middle Eastern bakers use it and it's amazing ground in with your espresso. Cardamom is a fave of Indian chefs too. It's often taken internally to help soothe occasional stomach discomfort. When you ingest it, Cardamom also promotes improved respiratory health with clear breathing. To top it off, its distinctive scent also promotes a positive mood. Amazing fragrance.

Cassia

This oil has been known to provide health benefits for thousands of years. Noted for its unique fragrance and calming aromatic properties, it's one of the few essential oils mentioned in the Old Testament. Feeling out of sorts? Cassia will promote healthy digestion and a healthy immune system when taken internally.

Cedarwood

Cedarwood is like a brisk walk in the forest. It not only promotes a feeling of wellness and vitality, it also helps your skin look healthy and acts as a natural insect repellant. Now that's multi-purpose! This oil is often used in massage therapy to create a relaxing atmosphere for the mind and body.

Clary Sage

This oil was a biggie in the Middle Ages. They used it to soothe the skin, and when you inhale Clary Sage it will help you feel relaxed and better able to get a good night's sleep. It's known for its calming properties, primarily because of linalyl acetate. It also promotes healthy-looking hair and is good for the scalp.

Douglas Fir

When anyone mentions Douglas Fir, visions of Christmas trees and snow-covered mountains immediately come to mind. It is a conifer that grows throughout North America. Douglas Fir's lemon-scented aroma is both sweet and refreshing, and its chemical makeup is especially rich in beta-pinene, which promotes a feeling of clear airways. It can be used to purify the skin and put you in a positive mood.

Frankincense

You have probably heard of Frankincense. One of my faves, this oil has definite biblical connotations, but it goes way beyond that. It helps reduce the appearance of skin imperfections and is generally rejuvenating and soothing. Sometimes referred to as the "king of oils," it can be used to help reduce the appearance of fine lines, wrinkles and skin imperfections. When taken internally, it supports healthy cellular function and its aroma sets the mood for feelings of relaxation.

EUCALYPTUS

If you live in California, you have definitely seen those beautiful eucalyptus trees towering over many of the other trees in your neighborhood. Eucalyptus trees are native to Australia. Also referred to as gum trees, Eucalyptus trees have definite properties that we use in our everyday lives. I use this oil to promote feelings of clear breathing and open airways. It's also helpful in creating a soothing massage experience. It's a multi-purpose oil that has purifying properties that can be beneficial for the skin.

FENNEL

Fennel is known for its distinct licorice aroma and taste, but it's also used to promote healthy digestion. The fennel plant can grow up to six feet tall and it's characterized by its delicate, feathery leaves. It was reportedly consumed by Roman warriors who used it to make them strong and prepared to do battle. Fennel is used to support the health of the lungs and respiratory tract. Others add it to water or tea to help fight sweet tooth cravings.

Fennel may help support the health of the lungs and respiratory tract and can be added to water or tea to help fight sweet tooth cravings. Fennel blends well with Basil,

Bergamot, Black Pepper, Cardamom, Cinnamon Bark, Cypress, Eucalyptus, Geranium, Grapefruit, Juniper Berry, Lavender, Lemon, Marjoram, Myrrh, Wild Orange, Patchouli, Rose, Rosemary, Sandalwood, Tangerine, and Ylang Ylang.

Geranium

Talk about diversity! There are more than 200 varieties of Pelargonium flowers, which are typically grown for their beauty, although just a few are used as essential oils. They're also a staple of the perfume industry. Back in Victorian times, fresh Geranium leaves were placed at formal dining tables as decorative pieces when people sat down for meals. Geranium oil was also once used by the ancient Egyptians to beautify their skin, among other benefits. I love it for calming nerves and reducing feelings of stress. Oh, and if you don't like bugs, it also repels insects.

Ginger

Ginger snaps and ginger ale are common remedies for an upset stomach. Now you can add Ginger essential oil to the list. When taken internally, Ginger is an effective digestive aid and it's good for helping to ease occasional indigestion and nausea. Ginger essential oil can also be applied topically or inhaled for a soothing aroma. Did you know you could also use it to help reduce bloating and gas?

Helichrysum

Okay, so Helichrysum may not be a fountain of youth, but it's often used to prevent signs of aging. That's pretty good, right? It's sometimes referred to as "The Everlasting Flower" because of its rejuvenating benefits for the skin and its ability to improve the complexion. It can help reduce the appearance of blemishes and it also promotes a glowing, youthful complexion.

Juniper Berry

Are you a gin lover? Gin comes from Juniper Berry. Personally, I'd rather use the oil. This all-round oil does a lot more than you'd expect. It supports healthy kidney and urinary tract function, serves as a natural skin toner and also acts as a natural cleansing and detoxifying agent. Beyond that, it has a calming, grounding effect on the soul. Just add one or two drops to water or citrus drinks and you've got a natural cleansing agent. Or apply one drop to promote a clear, healthy complexion. It can also be diffused with citrus oils to freshen and purify the air.

Lavender

And you knew I was not leaving Lavender off this list. This is one of the most popular essential oils because of its versatility. It has calming and relaxing properties that promote peaceful sleep and also ease feelings of tension. Applied topically, Lavender is often used to reduce the appearance of skin imperfections. You can also add it to bath water to soak away stress from a hard day, or you can apply it to the temples and the back of the neck for a relaxing experience.

Marjoram

Can I say, yummy? Known to the Greeks and Romans as a symbol of happiness, this oil has been used to spice up culinary dishes and it also adds a unique flavor to soups. Also known as "wintersweet," or "joy of the mountains," it's used in stews, dressings and sauces. In Germany this herb is known as the "Goose Herb" for its traditional use in roasting geese.

Marjoram is equally known for its calming properties and its positive effects on the nervous system when used internally. And if that wasn't enough, it supports both healthy cardiovascular and immune systems when taken internally. Marjoram can be used on surfaces throughout your house to protect against environmental threats. Or you can apply it to fingernails and toenails after showering. It keeps nails looking healthy.

Melissa

I love Melissa for so many reasons. It's pricey but worth every penny. This is a great all-round essential oil for reducing tense feelings, promoting relaxation and calming feelings of nervousness. Melissa officinalis, also known as lemon balm, was dubbed "Melissa" because of its sweet, fresh, citrus-like fragrance, which was known to attract bees. In fact, Melissa is Greek for "honey bee."

As one of the rarest and most expensive oils, Melissa can be used to flavor teas and ice cream (good excuse to have a scoop or two), as well as some fish dishes. Diffusing Melissa at night can also help you get a restful night's sleep.

Patchouli

If you like rich oils, Patchouli is one you'll love. With its rich, musky-sweet fragrance, Patchouli is regularly used by the perfume industry. It's also used for scented products like laundry detergents and air fresheners. Can you believe it's from the mint family? Patchouli is a bushy herb with stems reaching two or three feet in height and bearing small, pink-white flowers. It's beneficial to the skin, and when used topically, it helps to reduce the appearance of wrinkles, blemishes and minor skin imperfections. You can also apply it to the bottom of your feet for a calming effect.

Peppermint

Who doesn't like the fragrance or taste of Peppermint? I love it, especially with chocolate. Often used in toothpaste and chewing gum for oral hygiene, Peppermint also helps control occasional stomach upset and it's good for overall respiratory function when taken internally. And that fragrance? Place one drop in palm of your hand with one drop Wild Orange and one drop Frankincense and inhale for a wonderful pick-me-up.

Petitgrain

This oil's got a long history behind it, primarily for use in traditional health practices. Petitgrain essential oil is derived from the bitter orange tree and it's been used for cleaning purposes. But when taken internally, it supports a healthy immune system and nervous system function.

Roman Chamomile

Are you an insomniac? How would you like to get restful sleep while also getting support for healthy cardiovascular function and antioxidant support? Yes? Roman Chamomile is your perfect essential oil! It has a calming effect on the skin, mind and body, and may also help support healthy immune system function.

Hawaiian Sandalwood

This is another great oil that promotes healthy-looking, smooth skin while also reducing the appearance of skin imperfections. Hawaiian Sandalwood has a rich, sweet, woody aroma that instills calmness and well-being, making it a perfect oil to incorporate into massage or aromatherapy. It will also help to lessen tension in your life and promote emotional well-being.

Indian Sandalwood

This essential oil has a lovely fragrance that will enhance meditation and it's also very beneficial to the skin. It promotes healthy-looking, smooth skin and reduces the appearance of scars and other imperfections.

Sandalwood is a name given to a class of fragrant woods that, unlike other aromatic woods, can retain their fragrance for decades. Apply one to two drops to wet hair to help restore moisture and give hair a silky shine.

Vetiver

Vetiver is perfect for massage therapy! It can be rubbed on the feet before bedtime to promote a restful night's sleep. And when taken internally, Vetiver can support a healthy immune system. It promotes a calming, grounding effect on emotions and also has immune-supporting properties.

White Fir

White fir trees are a popular choice for Christmas trees. Native Americans used it as a building material because of its combination of strength, versatility, and beauty. White Fir essential oil is popular because it enhances feelings of soothing comfort.

Wild Orange

Want an energizing boost? I would not start my day without this oil. Just dispense one to two drops of Wild Orange in the palm of your hand and breathe deeply. It also blends well with other oils. Rub it on the back of your neck. It can be taken daily to cleanse the body or used on surfaces as a natural cleaner. How's that for versatility?

Ylang Ylang

Ylang Ylang has been used for centuries in religious and wedding ceremonies. Its essential oil is derived from the star-shaped flowers of the tropical Ylang Ylang tree and is used extensively in making perfumes and in aromatherapy. Ylang Ylang is frequently used in luxurious hair and skin products for its scent and nourishing and protective properties.

This is just a taste. Please check out Chapter Eleven for a list of recipes and blends you can use for cleaning, personal care and cooking. There are tons more on my blog; hayleyhobson.com/blog.

Chapter Nine

Cooking and Baking with Essential Oils

BY NOW you've learned that essential oils serve many purposes. And now we're on a topic I really love—cooking and baking with essential oils. Now, it goes without saying they benefit wellness. But did you know you could use them to enhance the flavor of your favorite recipes? Yes! You can! Many are so yummy.

I couldn't possibly write a book about essential oils without including this chapter on the culinary benefits of essential oils. There is more information available online, but I'll give you a jumpstart on which oils you can use with what types of foods when cooking and baking.

As you become more familiar with oils, you'll prepare your own blends. The best kind of container to use when mixing ingredients that contain essential oils is a glass or ceramic bowl. The oils could ruin certain types of plastic. And plastics contain toxins and chemicals. Why spoil your oil?

A common myth is that essential oils are expensive. It's true some are pricey, but you use so little that essential oils are a great value. They have a much longer shelf life than dried herbs or spices. You might spend a little more money up front but over time they will prove to be cost effective.

When creating blends and recipes, it's important that you don't drop the oil directly into your mixture because all essential oils tend to have different viscosity levels. Drop the required amount onto a spoon and then into your mixture to make sure you have the proper amount.

A common mistake people make when they start cooking or baking with essential oils is using too much. A little of these oils goes a long way, so it's best to add one drop, stir and taste. Repeat until you've reached your desired result.

Although essential oils are not poisonous, you'll want to store your oils out of reach of children. They're highly concentrated. And avoid touching the bottle inserts with your fingers because your natural oils could affect the oil composition.

Favorite Essential Oils for Baking and Cooking

Everyone has their personal faves. The list below contains some of the most popular and flavorful oils for cooking and baking. But make your own choices. I say, try them all and decide for yourself.

Ginger

Looking for a kitchen spice that's hot and earthy? This is it. The unique nature of Ginger adds flavor to lots of dishes and can help to support healthy digestion. Often used in Asian dishes, Ginger has a hot, fragrant flavor when used as a kitchen spice. In western tradition, Ginger is most often used in sweets. Gingerbread and ginger snaps are two examples. Use Ginger essential oil in your favorite sweet and savory dishes.

Do you like peanut butter cookies? Try the variation in Chapter Eleven.

Basil

The spicy, yet herbal nature of Basil makes it a versatile oil that can add extra flavor while cooking. Basil can be used to add a fresh, herbal flavor to meats, pastas and entrée dishes, and it's also cooling to the skin. The aroma of Basil helps promote a sense of focus and a stress-relieving experience. Add it to your scrumptious Italian dishes!

Peppermint

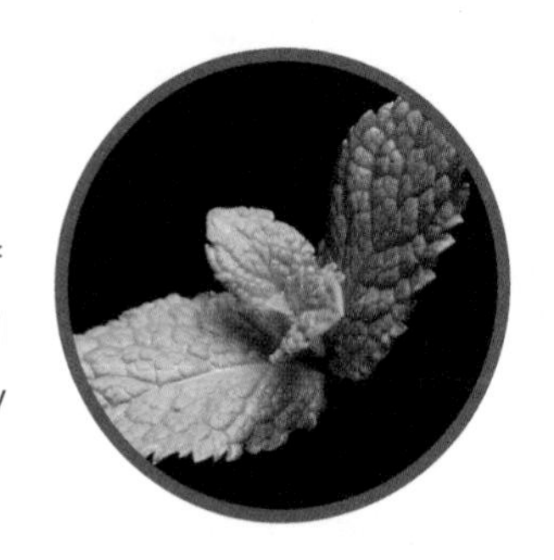

The Peppermint plant is a hybrid of Watermint and Spearmint. A high menthol content distinguishes the best quality Peppermint from other products.

Want to spice up your drinks? Just add a drop to your favorite smoothie recipe for a refreshing twist. Try a few drops in chocolate desserts or in Mediterranean salad dressings. And in hot chocolate.

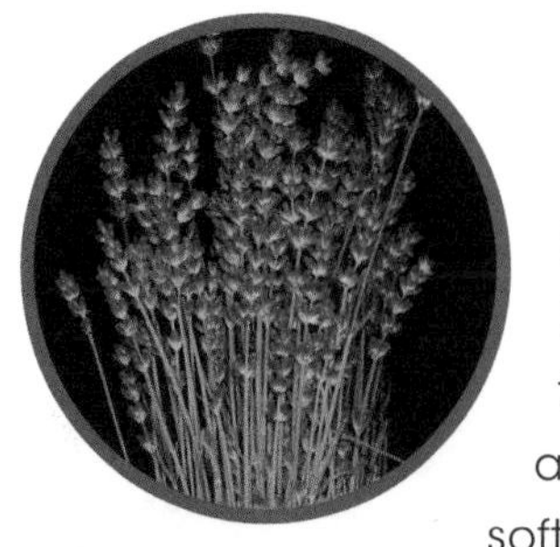

Lavender

Lavender again? Yep. You have to have it. Lavender has been used and cherished for centuries for its unmistakable aroma and myriad benefits. Use when cooking to soften citrus flavors and add a flavorful twist to marinades, baked goods, and desserts.

Lemon

Lemon is a great essential oil to have around. When added to water it provides a refreshing and healthy boost throughout the day. It's often added to food to enhance the flavor of desserts and main dishes. Taken internally, Lemon provides cleansing and digestive benefits and supports healthy respiratory function.

Lemongrass

Lemongrass is another versatile product. Its unique flavor has made it a favorite in Asian cuisine, as it's used in soups, teas and curries as well as with fish, poultry, beef, and seafood. Lemongrass essential oil promotes healthy digestion and acts as an overall tonic to the body's systems when ingested. It also blends well with Basil, Cardamom, or Spearmint.

Lime

Here's an essential oil that's both refreshing and energizing in aroma and taste. Limes are frequently used in entrées and beverages for their fresh, citrus flavor. A couple drops in your guacamole or in a baked chicken marinade is luscious. Due to its high limonene content, Lime also provides internal cleansing benefits.

Black Pepper

Want to add some kick to your cooking? Nothing works better than Black Pepper. With noted topical and internal benefits, Black Pepper essential oil can be used to ward off seasonal and environmental threats. It also aids in the digestion of foods, making it an ideal oil to cook with and enjoy both for its flavor and internal benefits. Add it to meats, soups, entrées and salads to enhance the flavor! It can be spicy so don't use too much.

Cardamom

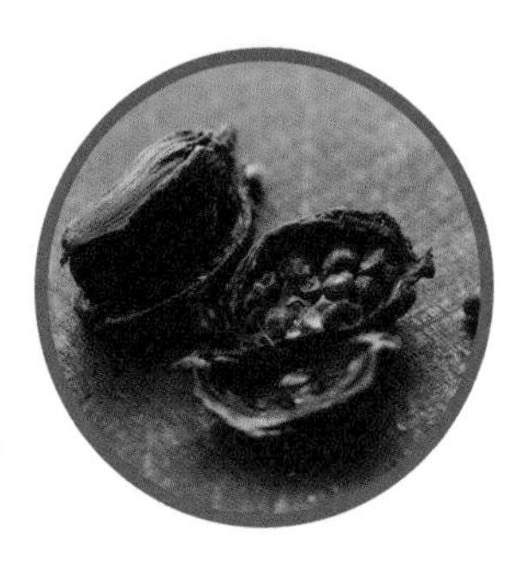

This is a close relative to Ginger. Although it's an expensive cooking spice, it is beneficial to the digestive system in a variety of ways. Add it to bread, smoothies, meats and salads to enhance food flavor and aid digestion.

Cilantro

This is big favorite for cooking—particularly in Mexican dishes. Cilantro's fresh, herbal aroma makes it perfect for cooking, while also providing powerful cleansing and detoxifying properties. The myriad uses and additional benefits of Cilantro have been documented for centuries. When taken internally, Cilantro promotes healthy digestion and supports healthy immune and nervous system functions. It can also add a flavorful twist to meats, salads, dips and guacamole. Add it to stir fries and salads to experience Cilantro's distinct flavor.

Cinnamon Bark

Cinnamon has a long history when it comes to culinary uses. It's derived from a tropical, evergreen tree that grows up to forty-five feet high and has highly fragrant bark, leaves, and flowers. Cinnamon oil, which is extracted from the bark, is a great overall health supplement. It supports healthy metabolic function and helps maintain a healthy immune system. It can also spice up desserts, entrées, and hot drinks!

Fennel

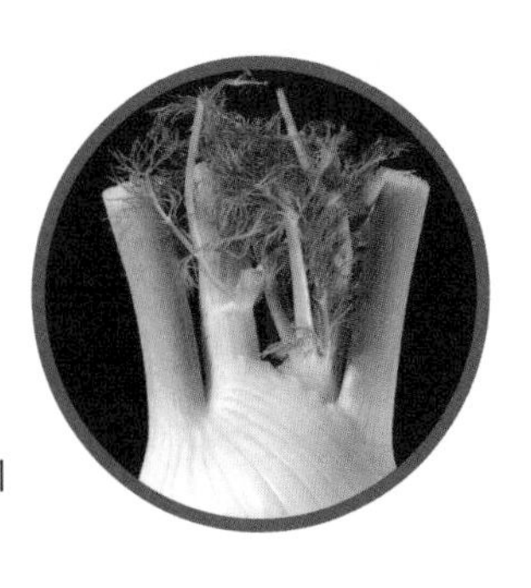

Fennel essential oil can still be used to promote healthy digestion and respiratory function, while producing a unique licorice aroma and flavor. You've gotta try the fennel salad recipe in Chapter Eleven.

Oregano

This one's been around for centuries and it's super versatile. It's one of the most potent and powerful essential oils and has long been used in traditional practices. The primary chemical component of Oregano is carvacrol, a phenol that possesses antioxidant properties when ingested. Put one drop in place of dried Oregano in spaghetti sauce, pizza sauce or on a roast. Mama Mia!

Rosemary

Rosemary is a multi-purpose essential oil that has loads of benefits. Its aromatic, evergreen shrub leaves are often used to flavor stuffings, pork, roast lamb, chicken, and turkey. It also supports healthy digestion and internal organ function. Keeps things moving—know what I mean?

Tasty foods really do enhance our experience of life. Using essential oils in your recipes provides a double benefit. Oils add flavor that makes our food taste good and they offer wellness benefits. Try some of the suggestions here or the recipes in Chapter Eleven, or experiment with your own.

Chapter Ten

Green Cleaning with Essential Oils

WHAT'S WITH all the hype about green cleaning? I mean seriously, does it really make a difference? Yes! And the impact is huge.

Why is green (also called eco-friendly) cleaning important? Well, first it's safer for you and your family than using cleaning products with chemicals. Green cleaning is also easy on the environment.

There are two myths I want to dispel right away:

Eco-friendly products don't work as well as chemicals.
They are super expensive.

Wrong on both counts. You'll never have to sacrifice quality because green products work just as well, if not better than chemical products. They are also affordable. In fact, making your own products actually saves money.

You probably already know this, but I'll say it anyway. Many of the household cleaners we use have toxic chemicals that can lead to health problems, whether short-term or long-term.

Hey! Want to hear something shocking? You know that nice, fresh smelling home you work hard to keep clean? Well, statistics from the U.S. Environmental Protection Agency reveal that the air inside an average home is 200 to 500 percent more polluted than the outside air, primarily because of all the cleaning products we use. Can you believe it? Makes you want to open a window, doesn't it?

Here's the worst part. The EPA says kids are especially vulnerable to the ill effects of chemicals during their formative years and it could even compromise their immune systems. It can also interfere with the development of their neurological, endocrine, and immune systems. Exposure can occur when they breathe fumes or touch the chemicals—not to mention when small children inadvertently eat or drink toxic cleaning products.

If you have toddlers, this is especially important. Younger children tend to inhale a bigger dose of the fumes from these chemicals because they have higher respiratory rates.

Your number one defense against a toxic lifestyle is to be prepared. Especially when it comes to cleaning supplies, we often reach for whatever's closest. Be sure to have the following basics on hand.

White Vinegar

This cuts grease and will dissolve those mineral deposits on your shower door. It also boasts natural antifungal and antibacterial properties. If you run out of white vinegar...get more. Save your Balsamic vinegar for your salads. It won't work the same.

Baking Soda

Oh yeah, it's a great all-purpose product. Sprinkle baking soda on the carpet, give it about fifteen minutes and then vacuum it up. Your carpet will look and feel fresh. You can also use baking soda to clean your sinks, bathtubs and countertops. It easily absorbs and eliminates unwanted odors.

Castile Soap

Castile soap is effective for cutting grease, lifting dirt, and getting rid of stubborn stains. You can also pour a small amount over your baking sheets and pans and scrub to get them looking shiny and new again. Try it!

Salt

It's not just for French fries. Believe it or not, this is an effective scouring agent. Mix some salt with hot water and pour it down your kitchen sink to remove unwanted odors and keep grease from building up. You can also remove coffee and tea stains by mixing salt with lemon essential oil.

Fractionated Coconut Oil or Olive Oil

Now here's a product that cleans effectively without toxic chemicals. You can rub it into your leather couch or use it to polish your wood furniture. All you need is a small amount.

How about a list of the most effective essential oils for cleaning? These eight oils are super powerful:

- Lemon
- Lime

- Douglas Fir
- Wild Orange
- Thyme
- Peppermint
- Melaleuca (Tea Tree)
- Eucalyptus

Here's a tip: ditch those toxic fake-smelling air fresheners and get a diffuser!

Onto the Blends!

You can create your own non-toxic cleaning products by mixing the following ingredients with essential oils. Here are some of the basics. Replace your chemical products with these.

Limescale Remover

Ingredients:

- 10 drops Lemon essential oil
- 10 drops Lime essential oil
- ½ cup baking soda
- 3 tablespoons water

Instructions:

1. Add water and essential oils to baking soda.
2. Mix into a paste.
3. Rub a small amount onto surface.
4. Let it sit for 20 minutes.
5. Wipe clean with a wet cloth.

Pine Floor Cleaner

Ingredients:

- 1 gallon of warm water
- 2 tablespoons of liquid castile
- 5 drops Cypress essential oil
- 5 drops White Fir essential oil
- 5 drops Douglas Fir essential oil
- 10 drops Lemon essential oil

Instructions:

1. Add soap and essential oils to a bucket of warm water.
2. Use a mop or rag to clean the floors.
3. Pour into spray bottle for cleaning countertops.

All-Purpose Cleaning Spray

Ingredients:

- 1 cup warm water
- 1 cup white vinegar
- 25 drops Wild Orange essential oil or other essential oil of your choice

Instructions:

1. Combine water and vinegar in a spray bottle.
2. Add essential oils of choice and shake vigorously.
3. Use on stainless steel, porcelain, wood, glass and countertops.
4. Wipe with a microfiber cloth or paper towel.

You might be nose blind but bet your guests can smell the odors in your house. Fish, broccoli, and your teenage athletes have distinctive odors.

STOP! Don't grab the bottles you have stored under the sink. The cleaning products most of us grew up with are petroleum based, toxic, or filled with ingredients we can't even spell. Throw those babies out.

Make your own eco-friendly cleaning products. Since you're just getting started using essential oils, I'll share some specific blends.

Eliminate Mold

You've probably heard about the dangers of mold. Add some tea tree oil to your diffuser and you've created an effective way to kill mold and other pathogens that may be drifting around in the air.

Carpet Cleaner

Pets and stinky feet can do a number on your carpet. How about a blend that will not only get your carpet smelling sweet, but also save you money in the process? Mix twenty drops of tea tree oil with Borax to create your own carpet powder.

Clean Kitchen Smell

Love fish but not the smell that lingers after cooking it? Get rid of all cooking odors by adding a few drops of clove, cinnamon or citrus essential oil to a simmering pan of water. It works!

Bathtub Scrub

None of us likes the discoloration and build-up that occurs in our bath tubs. But here's the remedy: mix one-half cup of baking soda, one-half cup of vinegar and five drops of Bergamot or lime oil. Then use the blend as a scrub for a sink or bathtub.

Sports Equipment Disinfectant

If your kids play soccer, baseball, or other sports, add three drops of lemon oil and three of tea tree oil to a few ounces of warm water. Use it to clean their sports equipment and gear.

Mosquito Repellent

Even if you're just hanging out in the back yard, this blend will keep those pesky skeeters away. Take it camping, to the beach and on picnics. Combine one drop of lemongrass oil, one drop of citronella oil and one drop of eucalyptus oil with a teaspoon of coconut oil. It creates a natural bug spray you can rub right on your skin.

All-purpose Cleaner

This blend is awesome! It works on a lot of surfaces. Add three drops each of Lemon oil and Tea Tree oil to a few ounces of warm water. Then spray your countertops and wipe with a clean rag to get rid of the germs.

Clean, Fresh Smelling Air

Cinnamon is one of the most fragrant elements. Grab your diffuser and a few drops of cinnamon essential oil. Then sit back, relax, and enjoy its anti-microbial properties.

Clean Burnt or Blackened Pans

Okay so, you know how blackened cooking pans can get, right? Lemon oil to the rescue! Add to boiling water to remove burnt food from pots and pans.

Yummy Smelling Home

This blend will overpower the odor from that stinky cat box or smelly kitchen trash can. Just diffuse clove, rosemary and orange essential oils when your guests come over. Instead of holding their noses, they'll be talking about how nice your home smells.

Washing Machine Cleanse

What's your favorite scent? Try This: add ten to twenty drops of essential oil (your choice) to every load. Your clothes will smell great!

Vacuum Cleaner

Deep six that dusty smell by adding five to ten drops of your favorite oil to your vacuum cleaner bag or dust container. Then just run the vac. Better yet, get one of the kids to do it!

Homemade Sunscreen

Here's a great one for the next time you're sitting poolside or hanging out at the beach. Mix coconut oil, zinc oxide, Shea butter, Helichrysum oil and Lavender essential oil. Then store it in a squeeze bottle for your next outing. Makes a great homemade toxic-free sunscreen.

Note: Coconut oil has an SPF of around seven. That's NOT enough protection for fair-skinned folks or kids. Non-burning UVB rays can also cause serious long-term damage to skin. For best results, limit your time in the sun.

Shower Curtain Scum

There's nothing more annoying than the discoloration that accumulates on your shower curtain. But here's a solution: take a sixteen ounce spray bottle and mix four drops of eucalyptus essential oil and four drops of tea tree oil (melaleuca) with warm water. Then simply spray it onto your shower curtain to kill the mold.

Kill Pests

My rules for bugs: your house, your rules, my house, my rules. Want a quick and easy way to keep ants and other bugs at bay? Spray a mixture of Wild Orange essential oil and clove oil to kill those pests on contact.

Fresh Trash Can

Trash cans are the source of some of the worst kitchen odors. Here's the remedy: put a cotton ball with two drops each of Lemon oil and Tea Tree oil at the bottom of the trash. It will decrease the odor and detoxify the air.

Bathroom Freshener

Talk about quick and easy! Place a cotton ball soaked in Lime or Lemon oil behind the toilet for an effective and green bathroom refresher.

Purify the Fridge

Here's another area that can generate unwanted food odors. And boy do they rush out at you when you open the fridge. To freshen the fridge or freezer when cleaning, add a few drops of Lime, Grapefruit or Bergamot oil to the rinsing water.

Eliminate Smoke

Live with a smoker? Few things linger like the smell of cigarette or cigar smoke. To get rid of it, put four drops of Rosemary, Tea Tree, and Eucalyptus oil in a spray bottle and spray around the house. And then ask the smoker to please step outside from now on.

Sparkling Dishes

Okay, here's a simple way to get your dishes looking spot-free. Just add a few drops of Lemon oil with detergent to the dishwasher before washing.

Smelly Shoes

Feet sweat. Sweat stinks. Here's a blend a lot of people could use. Add a few drops of Tea Tree oil and Lemon oil to freshen those shoes and remove unwanted odors.

The fact that homes and buildings are better insulated than ever before holds in toxins. Keep your windows open as often as possible to allow fresh air in and allow toxins to flow out. This is especially important when cleaning your home.

If you don't have time to clean your own home, fortunately there are a ton of green cleaning services out there to help scour and scrub for you. Call around and ask what types of cleaning products are used.

If you can't find one in your area, don't be shy! Find a service willing to use your blends or products and methods you prefer.

If your housekeeper doesn't use green products, make your own and ask him or her to use them. There's no reason not to rid your life of toxic cleaning products.

Chapter Eleven

Some of My Favorite Recipes and Blends

HERE WE are, on our final lap. If you've read the first ten chapters of my book, I would say you have a pretty good background on essential oils. You know when and why to use them, what their unique properties are, and how they can enhance your life.

Use what you learned to discover which oils you like best and which address your specific wellness concerns. Most of all, have fun.

Soon you'll be creating recipes and blends of your own, and to get you started, I'm passing along some of my personal faves. I've included blends for cleaning, cooking and personal care.

Concentration

Essential oils are highly concentrated. One drop might be all you need and even that might need to be diluted in water or carrier oils like fractionated coconut oil or almond oil. Don't think that just because you use more than suggested you will have greater benefits. You need only a small amount. Use accordingly.

Not all essential oil companies sell pure oils. I use oils that are certified pure therapeutic grade (CPTG). They are free from additives and dilutions. Always research companies before you buy oils from them.

Some oils can be taken internally, others cannot. Keep learning and be aware. Just because essential oils are natural doesn't mean you don't treat them with respect.

Photosensitivity

Certain oils can make your skin more sensitive to the sun. Citrus oils are the ones to watch out for if you're planning to spend the day hiking or at the beach. If you do apply essential oils to your skin, wait a minimum of four to five hours before exposing yourself to UV rays. NEVER use oils topically when tanning.

Pregnant or Nursing

ALWAYS ask your doctor before using essential oils. Some are considered safe and others can be dangerous during pregnancy. Some can cause a dangerous hormonal imbalance.

The National Association for Holistic Aromatherapy (NAHA), recommends that pregnant women avoid the following essential oils:

- **Wintergreen essential oil**
- **Sage essential oil**
- **Mugwort essential oil**
- **Tarragon essential oil**
- **Birch essential oil**
- **Aniseed essential oil**
- **Camphor essential oil**
- **Hyssop essential oil**
- **Parsley essential oil (seed or leaf)**
- **Pennyroyal essential oil**
- **Tansy essential oil**

- **Thuja essential oil**
- **Wormwood essential oil**

If you're nursing, it might also be best to avoid Peppermint essential oil as it can decrease milk supply. But...if you're in the process of weaning, that can be helpful! Ask your doctor if you can use Peppermint topically on the breasts.

Drug Interaction

If you're taking prescription medication, some essential oils have been known to interact, so again, ask your doctor before using oils. And if you suffer from liver or kidney disease, or if you have a compromised immune system, some doctors suggest you not use essential oils at all. Others say oils are fine. Always ask.

Kids and Essential Oils

As I've said, children can benefit from using oils, but there are a few things to remember. Children have thinner skin than adults. They are extremely sensitive to potency, so dilute essential oils at least double what you would for an adult.

-

And now...your Blends and Recipes!

Diffuser Blends

The best diffusers aren't always the most expensive ones, but the ones that do the best job. Here are the most common varieties.

Nebulizers are the most powerful and don't require heat or water.

Ultrasonic diffusers are similar to nebulizers except they require water.

Evaporative diffusers cause oils to evaporate when dropped on a pad or filter and blown by a fan.

Heat diffusers are similar to evaporative but use heat instead of a fan.

Just remember, buy a diffuser that performs. If you go cheap, what you save on the diffuser will be spent in wasted efficiency and squandered oils.

Try these diffuser blends....

Wake Up

Are you a morning person? No? These blends will help you wake up refreshed even before you head for the coffee! I swear! They're ideal to evoke a sense of focus and positive mood first thing in the morning.

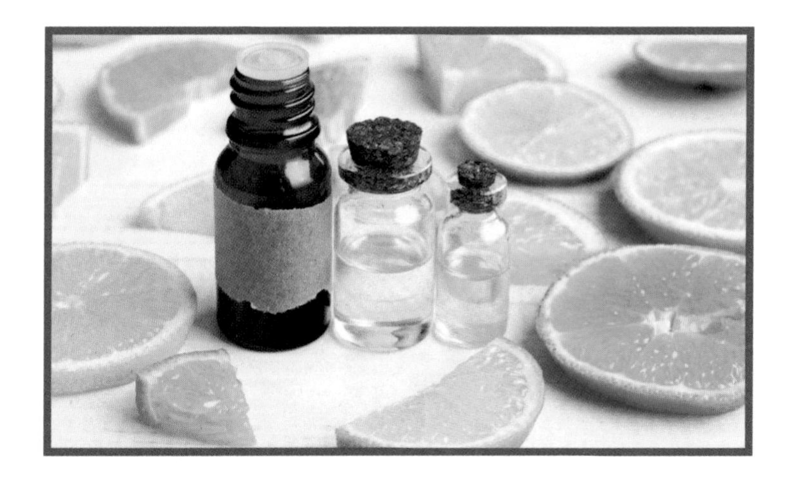

- 2 drops each
- Lime
- Lemon
- Wild Orange
- Grapefruit
- Bergamot

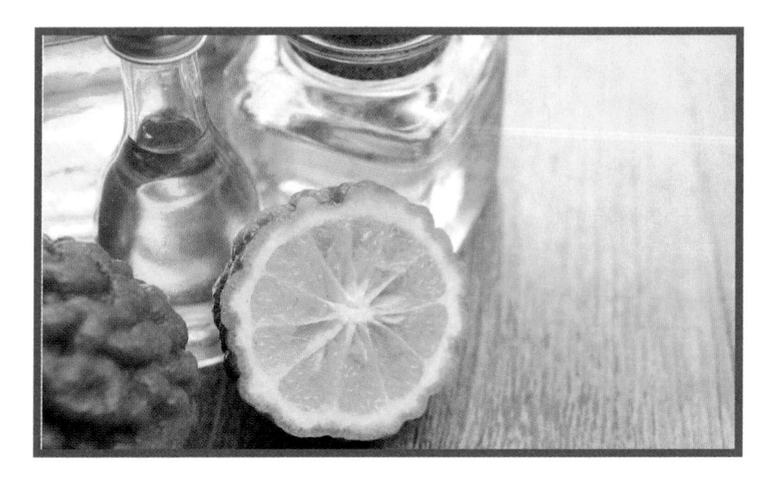

- 5 drops Bergamot
- 3 drops Grapefruit
- 2 drops Peppermint

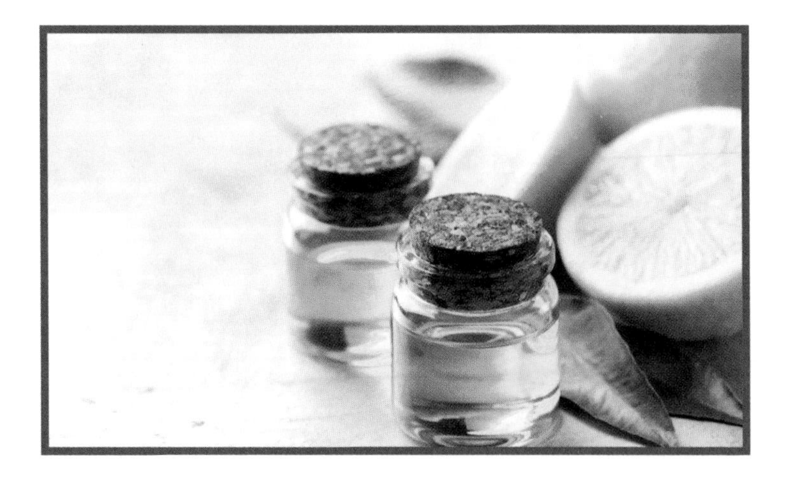

- 4 drops Lemon
- 2 drops Lime
- 3 drops Melaleuca

Peaceful Sleep

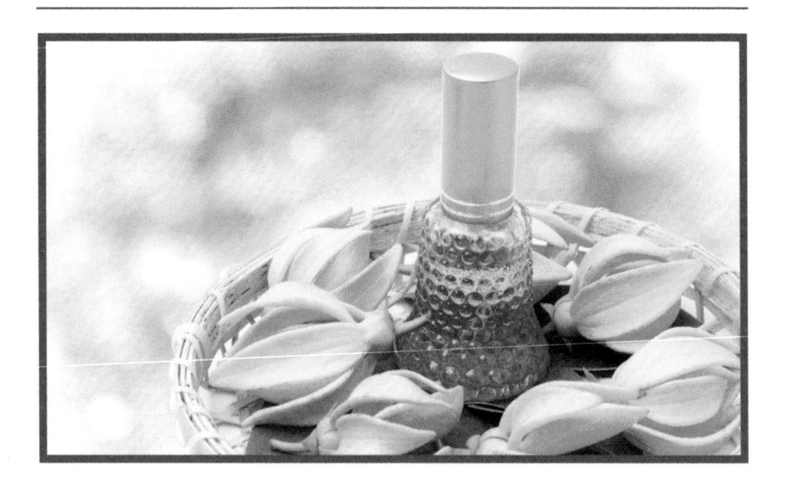

Do you have trouble settling in after a long day? Does your mind keep reeling as thoughts become broken records? Try this blend and sleep quietly and peacefully. Catch those Z's!

- 4 drops Lavender
- 2 drops Ylang Ylang

Tension Release

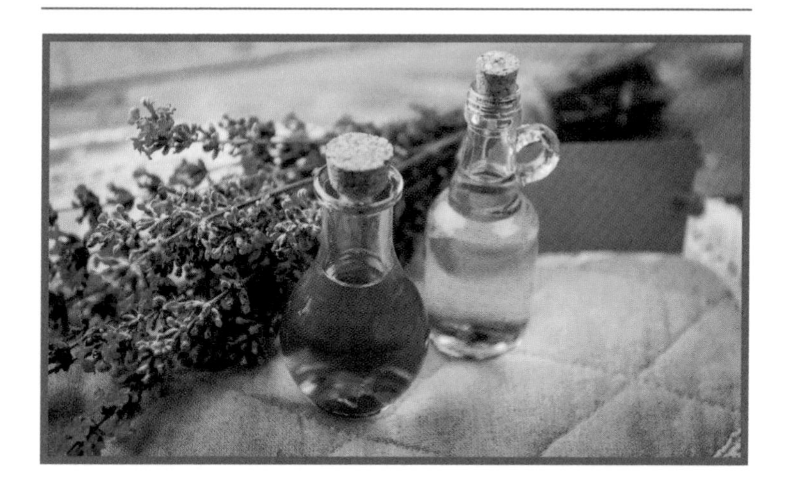

Stress and tension are the cause of mental distress and physical disease. This blend will help bring relief.

- 3 drops Lavender
- 3 drops Clary Sage
- 2 drops Ylang Ylang
- 1 drop Marjoram

Sadness

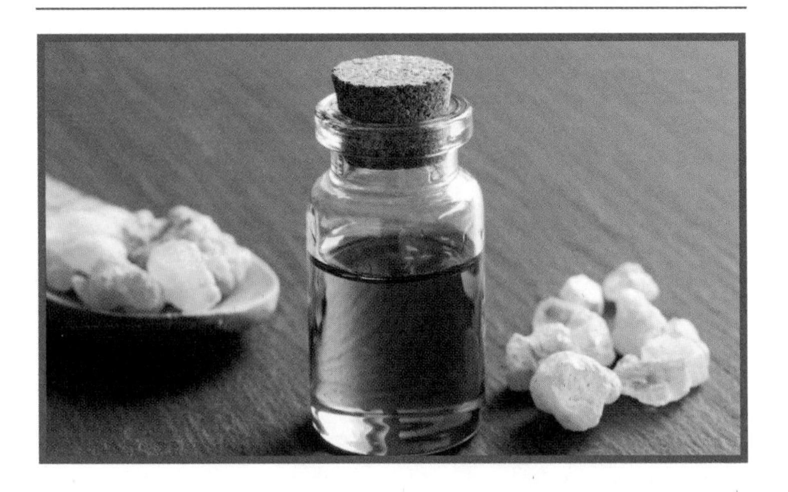

Even though sadness is a natural emotional response it can be debilitating at times. Use this blend to help lift your spirits when you're feeling down in the dumps.

- 2 drops Bergamot
- 2 drops Frankincense

Relax and Reconnect

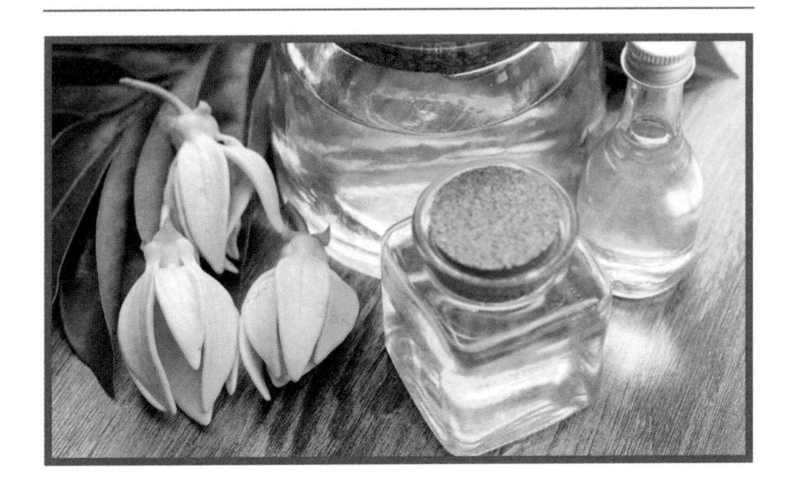

My husband, Wes, and I love to travel for pleasure and we also travel for business. We love spending a few days alone with each other and we use this blend to help us relax and connect.

- 2 drops Lavender
- 2 drops Ylang Ylang

Add to your diffuser to ease tension and reduce anxiety.

Self-Confidence

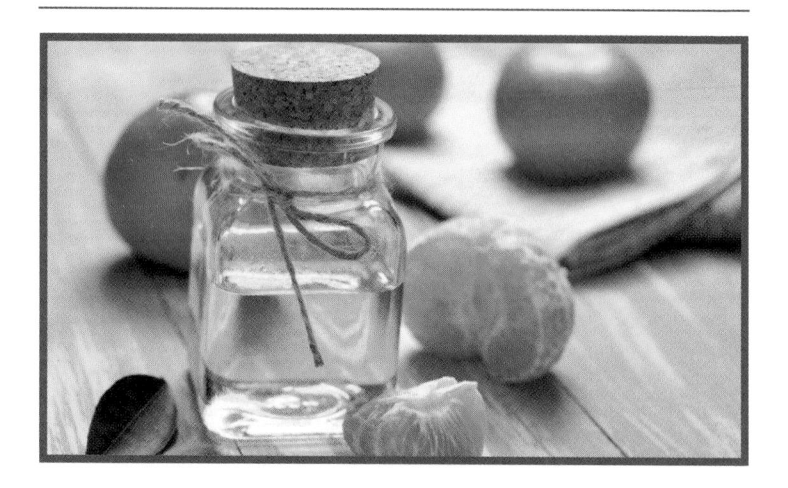

I diffuse this blend to help promote feelings of being powerful and belief in my self. Got a big presentation to do? Or even a mini one? Feeling like you need a confidence boost? Wild Orange energizes and uplifts the mind and body while purifying the air.

- **5 drops Elevating Blend (Lavender, Sandalwood, Tangerine, Melissa, Ylang Ylang, Lemon)**
- **3 drops Wild Orange**

Moving Through Fear

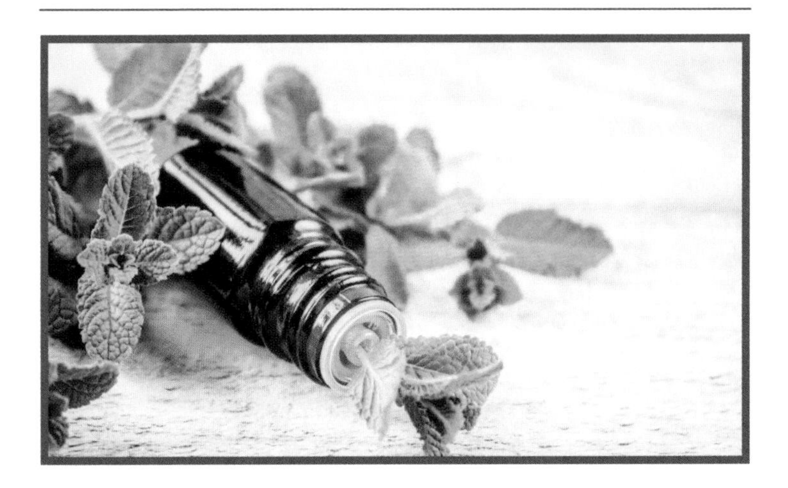

Fears and obstacles can prevent all of us from moving forward by keeping us stuck. And you probably know if you want to write a new chapter in your life, you're going to have to find that way to move through the obstacles in front of you (or that you may even be self-imposing) so you can get on. This blend can help you move through that fear you may be having.

- 2 drops Sandalwood or Roman Chamomile
- 2 drops Frankincense
- 2 drops Peppermint

Focus

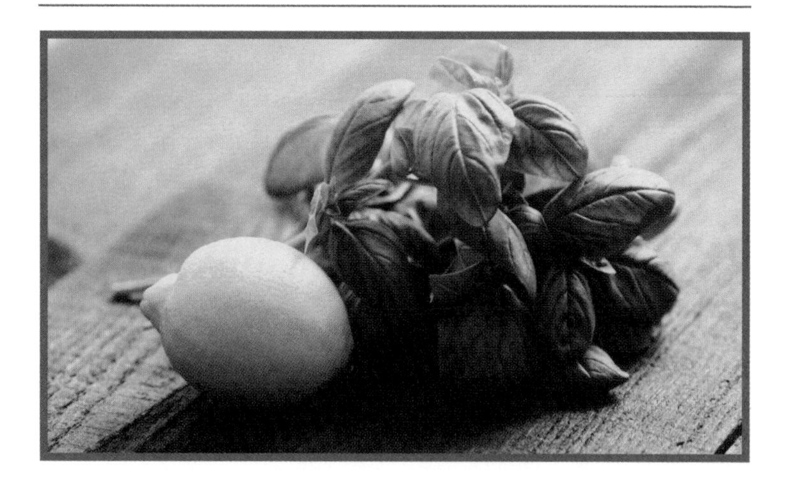

Try this blend when you need to be alert and energized. At your desk, in front of your computer, in an important conversation, or even when you're running around with your littles. It also promotes a positive mood. It's your secret recipe to get things done!

- 1 drop Douglas Fir
- 1 drop Basil
- 2 drops Lemon

Concentration and Energy

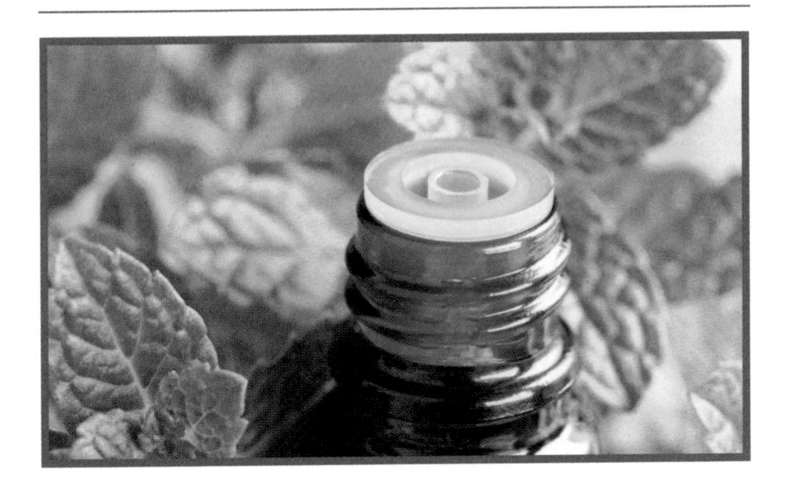

Does your mind wander? OMG, mine does for sure! I've got to stay laser focused in order to get everything done so I use this to help maintain concentration.

- 2 drops Peppermint
- 1 drop Rosemary

Push Your Limits

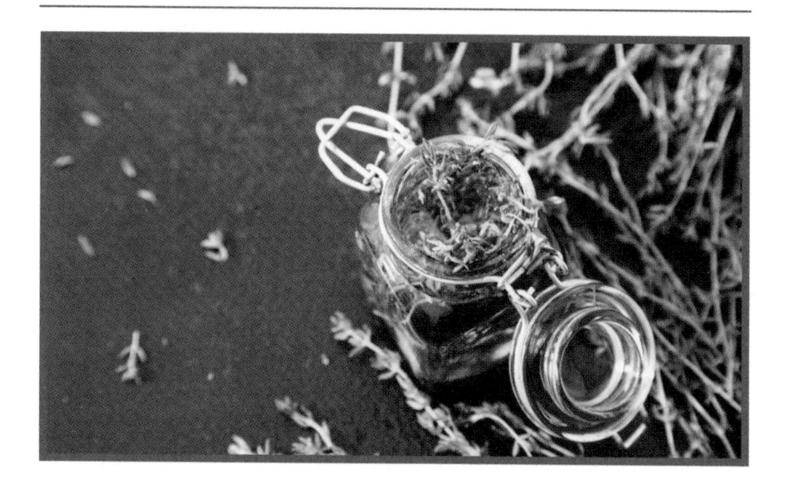

We all need that extra push now and then. Especially at the end of the day when we still have work to do. This blend will help perk you right up!

4 drops each:

- Black Pepper
- Thyme
- Wild Orange
- Frankincense

Positive Attitude

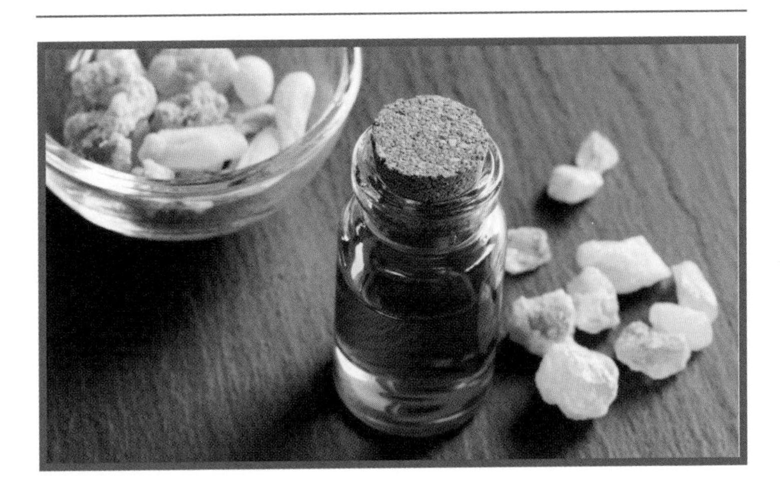

Ready to recharge and relax. Lavender will help reduce any anxious feelings you may be having and Wild Orange will uplift your body and mind. As if that weren't good enough already, Ylang Ylang promotes a positive outlook.

3-4 drops each:

- Frankincense
- Lavender
- Ylang Ylang

Relax and Uplift your Mood

Bergamot oil can help promote uplifting, relaxing, and confident feelings—particularly when diffused. When diffusing on its own, use three to four drops of Bergamot oil in the diffuser of your choice. Diffusing this oil can help promote a sense of self-confidence when you feel frazzled, or a sense of inner peace when feelings of stress abound.

Motivation

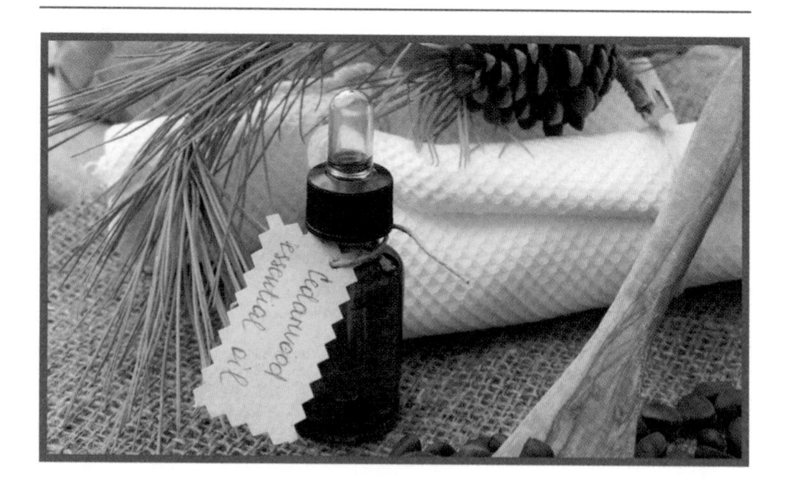

This blend will help you get up and get going, set goals and make clear decisions. You gotta love that, right?

2 drops Each:

- Cedarwood
- Frankincense
- Grapefruit
- Lemon
- Juniper Berry
- Black Pepper

My Favorite Morning Blend

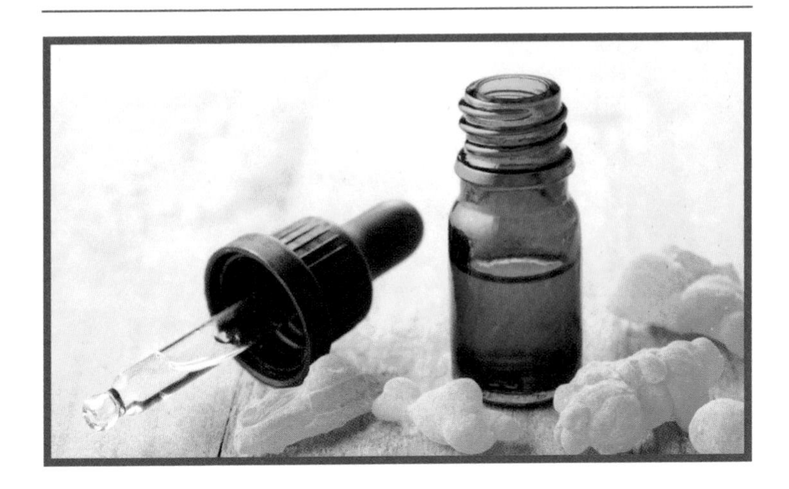

Let's be honest, sometimes it's hard to wake up in the morning and really get going. Especially Mondays! I love this blend. Mix it with fractionated coconut oil and apply all over your body!

2 drops Each:

- Wild Orange
- Frankincense

Here's my personal plan of attack against jet lag and brain fog. Check out these blends.

What Jet Lag?

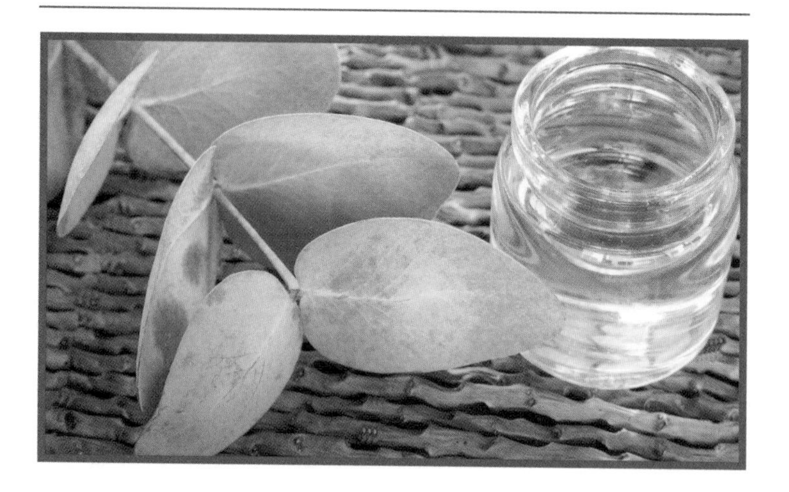

5 drops Each:

- Citrus Bliss
- Wild Orange
- Bergamot
- Peppermint
- Eucalyptus

Train Your Body Clock

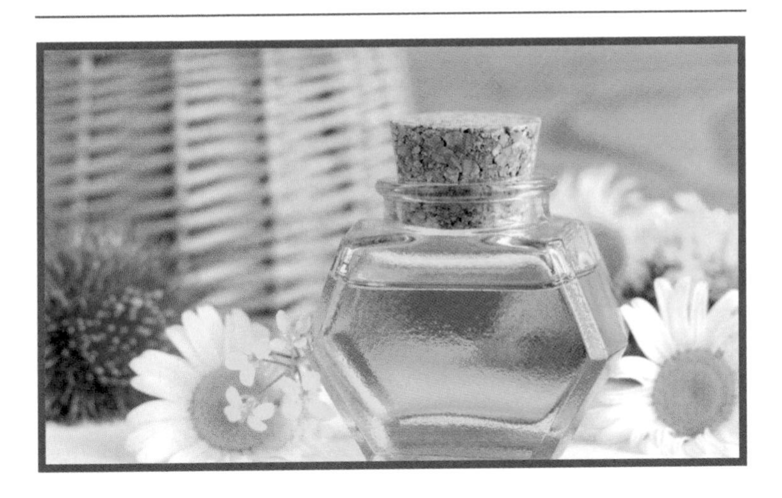

5 drops Each:

- Roman Chamomile
- Lavender
- Sweet Marjoram

Erase Travel Funk

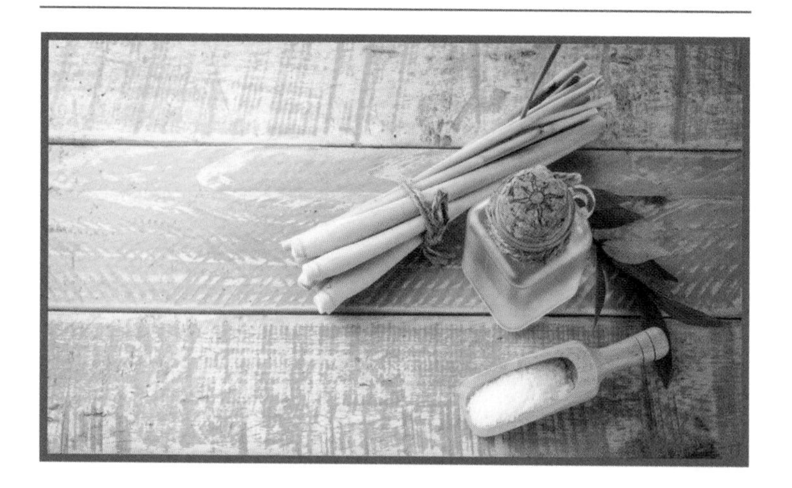

2 drops Each:

- Citrus Bliss
- Lemongrass

Immune Booster

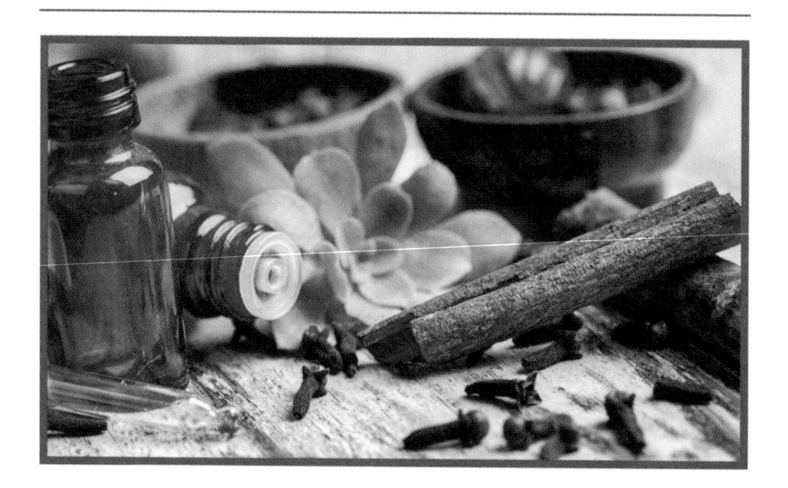

In need of an immune booster? Who isn't, right? You don't need an excuse to stay strong and healthy all year round. Use a rollerball bottle and apply this blend to your feet or the sides of your spine.

5 drops Each:

- Frankincense
- Wild Orange
- Eucalyptus
- Cinnamon

WEEKEND CHILL

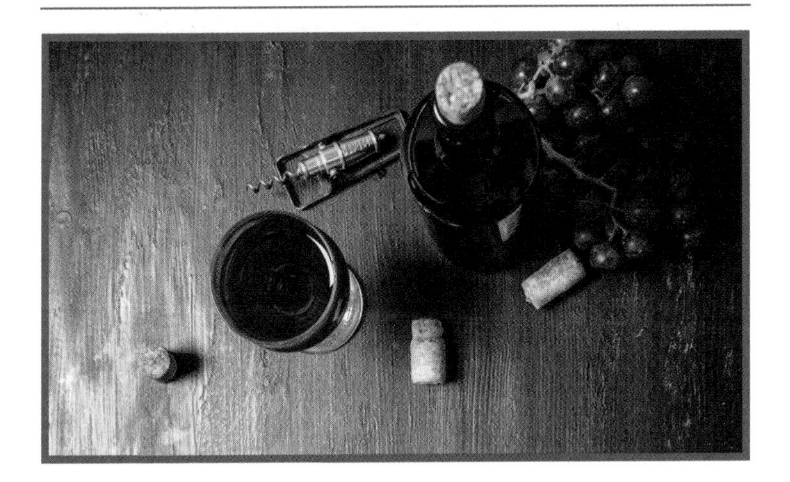

This is an awesome diffuser blend to get you nice and relaxed after a stressful day or week. Actually, you don't need to have a stressful day or week. It's an amazing blend no matter what!

- 3 drops Grapefruit
- 2 drops Orange
- 2 drops Lemon

- 1 drop Bergamot
- 1 Glass of Wine (optional)

Uplift

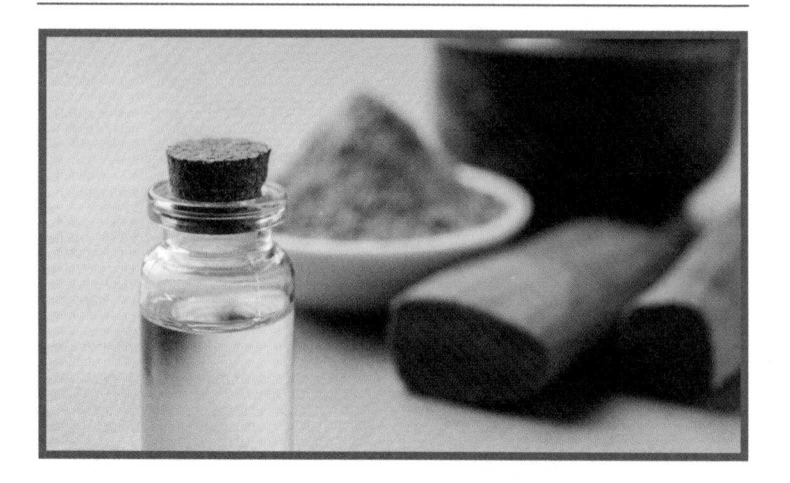

Diffuse this blend to uplift your mind, body and soul. It's a global pick-me-up for your entire body.

- 4 drops Eucalyptus
- 2 drops Grapefruit
- 2 drops Ylang Ylang or Sandalwood

Happy Mom Blend

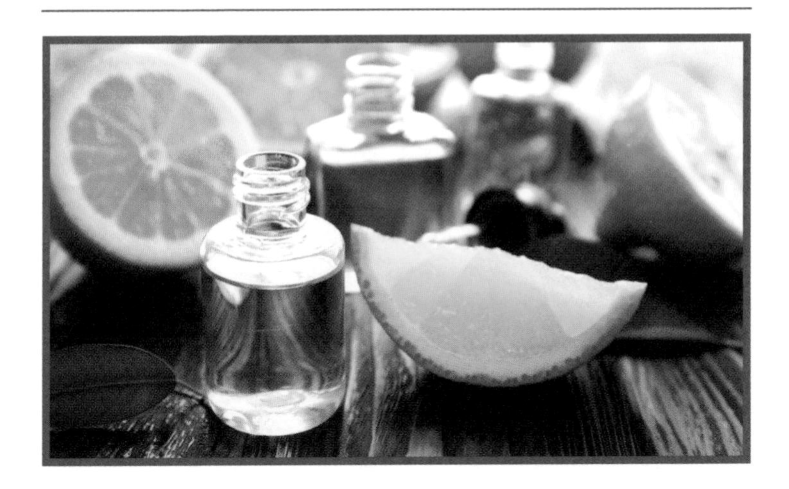

This diffuser blend should help relieve the stress, help find clarity, create calming thoughts and a happy environment. A happy mom is a happy home. Enjoy!

- 2 drops Wild Orange
- 2 drops Bergamot

PARADISE

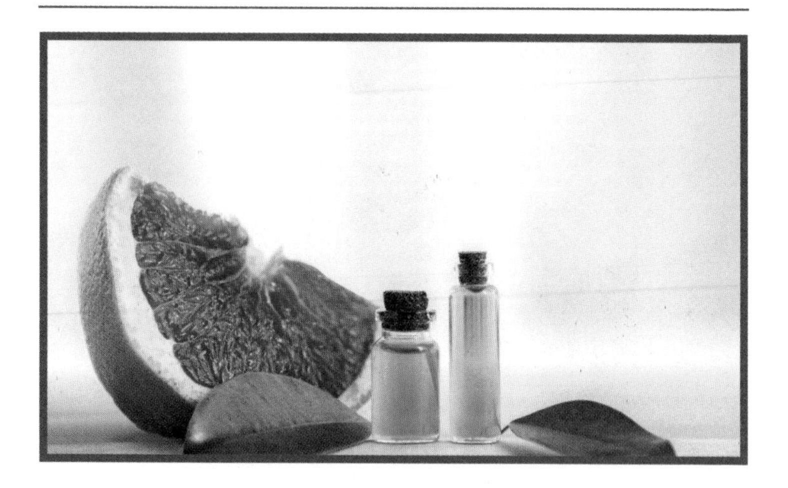

Summer sandals and citrus all wrapped up in a diffuser blend! You don't have to go all the way to the Bahamas to experience paradise. You will love this!

- 3 drops Citrus Bliss
- 2 drops Sandalwood
- 3 drops Grapefruit

Morning Blend

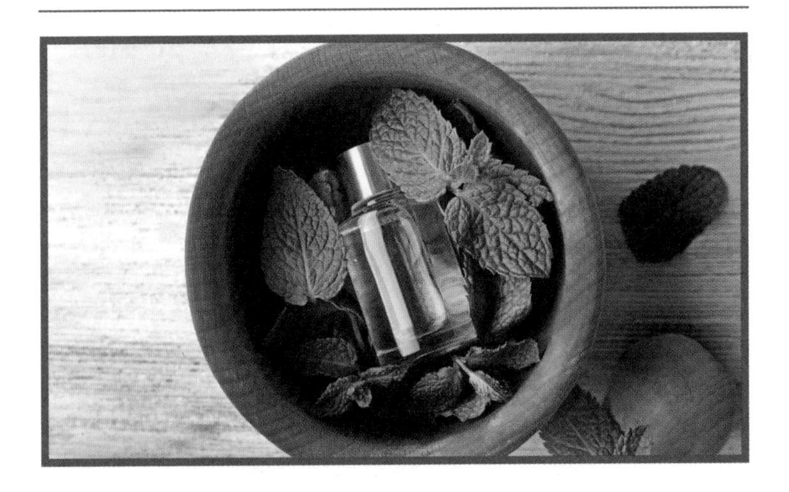

Try this refreshing blend first thing in the morning to clear out the brain fog and start your day with the right mindset. These are all great oils to lift your mood and invigorate your mind!

- 3 drops Peppermint
- 2 drops Spearmint
- 1 drop Wintergreen

CLEANING BLENDS

FRESHENING SPRAY

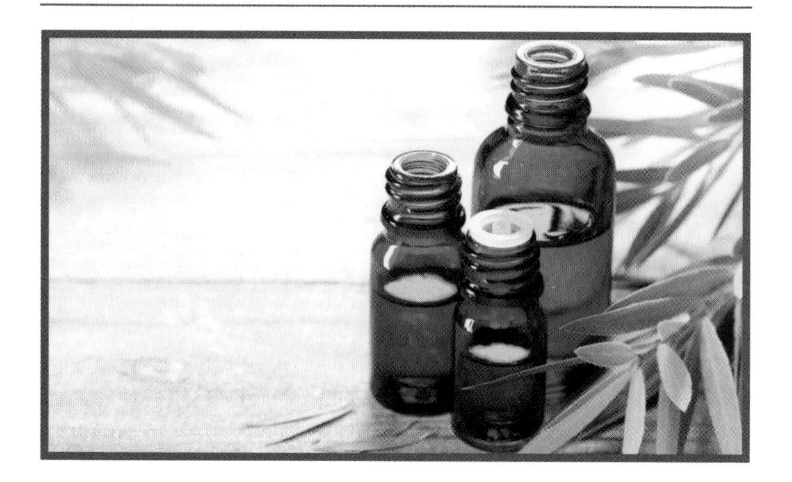

If your morning or evening routine includes wiping down the counters, this blend is fresh and fragrant. Add it to your cleaning arsenal. It purifies the air from foul odors and is an effective cleaner.

Ingredients:

- 2 drops Siberian Fir Needle
- 2 drops Citronella Grass
- 2 drops Lime
- 2 drops Lemon
- 3 drops Melaleuca (tea tree oil)
- 2 drops Cilantro

My three favorite ways to use it around the house are:

Add 5 drops to a small spray bottle with water and use to wipe down my counter tops.

Freshen my car and different rooms of the house, by placing a few drops on a cotton ball and putting them into an air vent or using a car diffuser.

Diffuse around my house as I'm cleaning to purify and freshen the air. Way better than the popular chemical spray!

Dish Soap

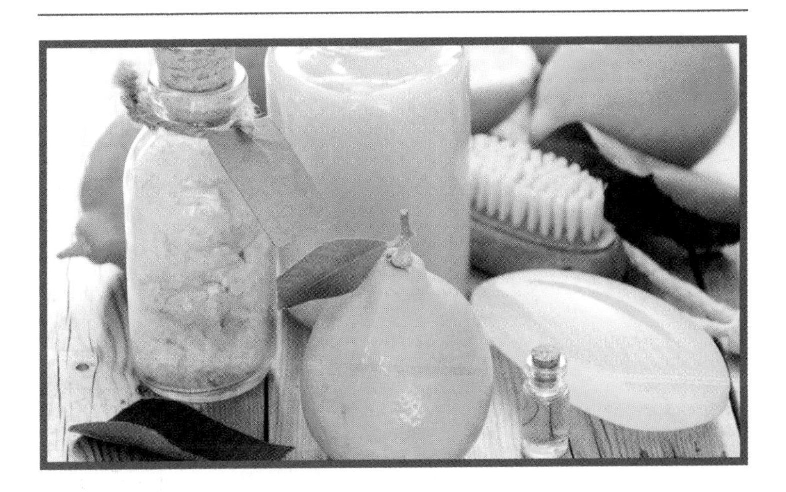

This smells great and cleans your dishes well!

Combine 2 cups of castile soap with:

- 20 drops Lime
- 8 drops Lemon
- 6 drops Citrus Bliss

PERSONAL CARE

BODY BUTTER

I'm OBSESSED with skin care! And now I'm giving you a recipe you can do yourself at home. I got this from an essential oils blog. The butter and oils used in this blend will leave your skin moisturized for days after applying.

Customize *your* body butter with the essential oil of your choice. Some of my favorites are:

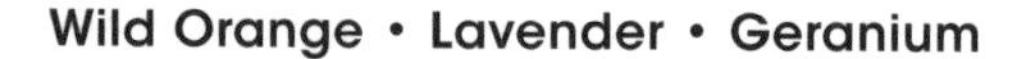

Wild Orange • Lavender • Geranium

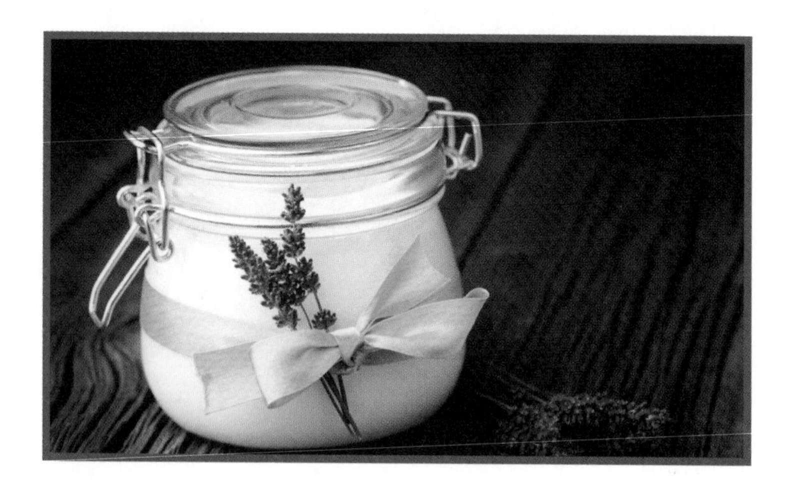

Ingredients:

- ½ cup Shea Butter
- ½ cup Cocoa Butter
- ½ cup Fractionated Coconut Oil (You can also use almond oil)

- 15 drops Grapefruit essential oil
- 15 drops Wild Orange essential oil
- Double Boiler, Hand Mixer

Instructions:

1. Measure all of the butters and oils into glass jar.
2. Fill a large skillet or saucepan with 1–1.5 inches of water. Bring to a boil. Once boiling, add the glass jar to the center of the saucepan to melt and combine ingredients.
3. Stir every few minutes until the ingredients are melted and combined (10–15 minutes).

Tip: Use a Popsicle stick to stir for easy cleanup.

4. Once everything is melted, remove from heat and let sit for 5–10 minutes. Add desired essential oils.
5. Once essential oils are added, let it rest in a cool place (such as the refrigerator) until it has set.
6. Once chilled, take out of refrigerator. With a stand or hand mixer, start on low and slowly turn the speed higher until the lotion becomes light and fluffy (around 3–5 minutes).
7. You're done! Store mixture in a glass jar and keep in a cool place. You can re-fluff the body butter by simply whipping it back up with a hand mixture to the consistency you prefer.
8. This whipped body butter makes a great gift and can easily be customized by using your choice of essential oils. The options are endless!

Detangler

This is one of my favorite DIY recipes, especially during the summer! Pool hair can be the worst. Try this detangler blend right after you get out of the shower, before you brush your hair. You will feel the difference immediately. Enjoy no more tangles!

Ingredients:

- 1 cup Distilled Water
- 1 tsp. Grape Seed Oil
- 2 tsp. Fractionated Coconut Oil
- 10 drops Citrus Bliss Essential Oil

Instructions:

Spray onto hair and brush through.

Improve Cellulite

I finally found a great solution to cellulite with this amazing essential massage oil blend. Cellulite is caused by fluid retention, lack of circulation, weak collagen structure and increased body fat.

This blend of oils will improve circulation and flush out toxins and fats naturally!

- Spruce needle/leaf
- Ho wood
- Frankincense
- Blue Tansy Flower
- Blue Chamomile Flower
- Fractionated Coconut Oil

Stiffness and Tightness

No one wants to feel the kinks and cranks in their body. Instead, we all prefer to keep ourselves in top shape and ready to go each day, right? Try this blend and notice how great you feel.

- 1 drop Black Pepper
- 1 drop Bergamot
- 2 drops Frankincense
- 2 drops White Fir
- Fractionated Coconut Oil

Mouthwash

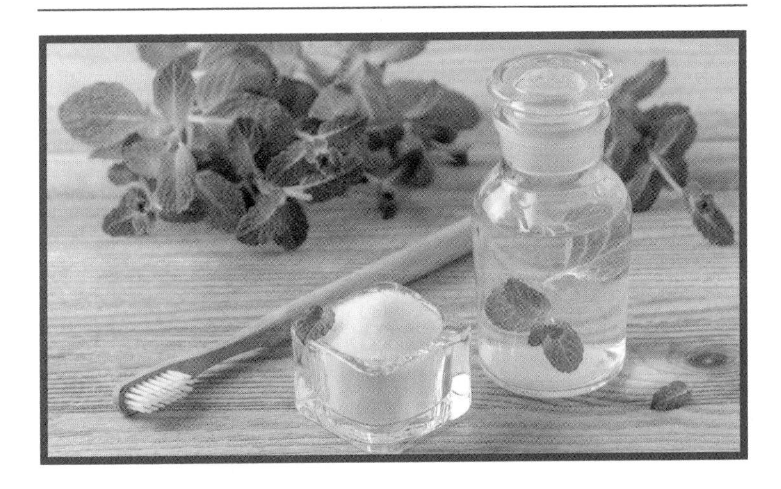

You can use either Peppermint or Spearmint essential oil, with both being great for oral care. Spearmint is the milder option. Myrrh is included for its cleansing properties, especially for its ability to cleanse the mouth and throat.

NOTE: Remember that essential oils don't stay mixed in water based formulations, so it's necessary to shake the mouthwash well before every use. Otherwise use it as any other mouthwash!

- 6 oz. Water
- 8 drops Peppermint or Spearmint
- 5 drops Myrrh

FOOD AND BEVERAGE RECIPES

Gluten-Free Pancakes

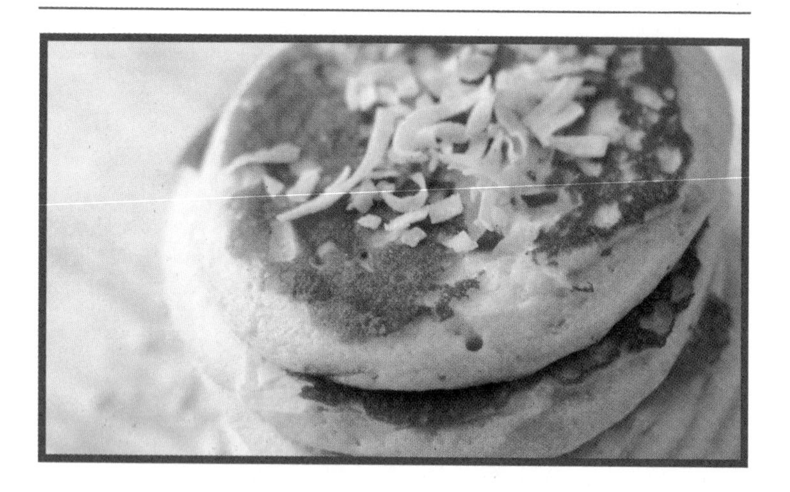

Ingredients:

- 4 eggs (Organic Free Range) or Egg Substitute
- 4 tbsp of Coconut Flour
- 1-2 drops Cinnamon Bark Essential Oil
- 1 drop Wild Orange (optional)
- Unsweetened Coconut Flakes (to sprinkle on)

- ¼ cup Coconut Milk or Almond Milk
- 1 tsp organic vanilla extract

NOTE: Vary the amount of flour or milk depending on how you like your pancakes.

Instructions:

1. Mix all ingredients in a bowl and then let it all settle for a few minutes.
2. Heat up your pan and add olive oil or your choice of oil.
3. Add pancakes mixture pan—start small until you get the hang of your batter mix.
4. Cook each side until it bubbles and is easy to flip. Because this isn't regular flour it can take a little longer to cook.
5. Top your cooked pancakes with your unsweetened coconut, maple syrup, bananas and berries or whatever you choose.

Dark Chocolate Detox Bites

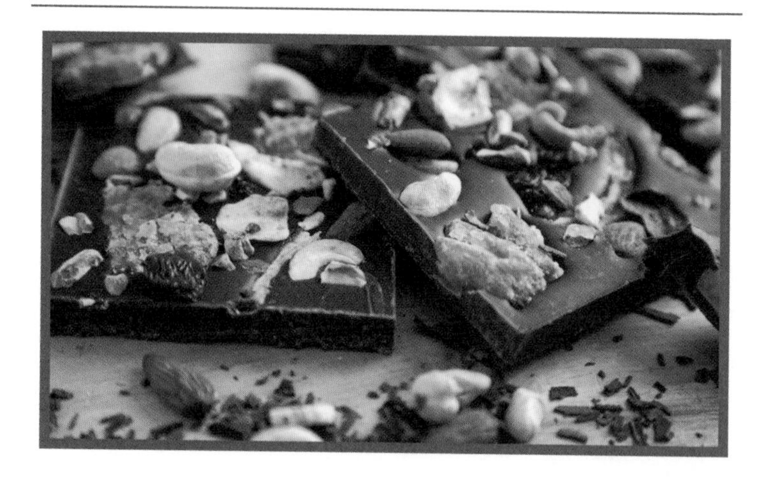

These simple healthy Dark Chocolate Detox Bites will revolutionize your dessert habits! Not only do you get to indulge your chocolate addiction, but this helps detox the body at the same time.

Peppermint and Grapefruit oil have been shown to improve bloating, dissolve fat, cravings, and digestion.

Ingredients:

- Assorted Dried Fruits and Nuts
- 1 drop Grapefruit or Peppermint essential oils
- 8 oz. Dark Chocolate

Instructions:

1. Melt chocolate over stove.
2. Stir in essential oils until there are no lumps.
3. Drop rounds of chocolate onto parchment paper.

4. Sprinkle healthy add-ins on top while chocolate is still hot.
5. Refrigerate.

Guacamole

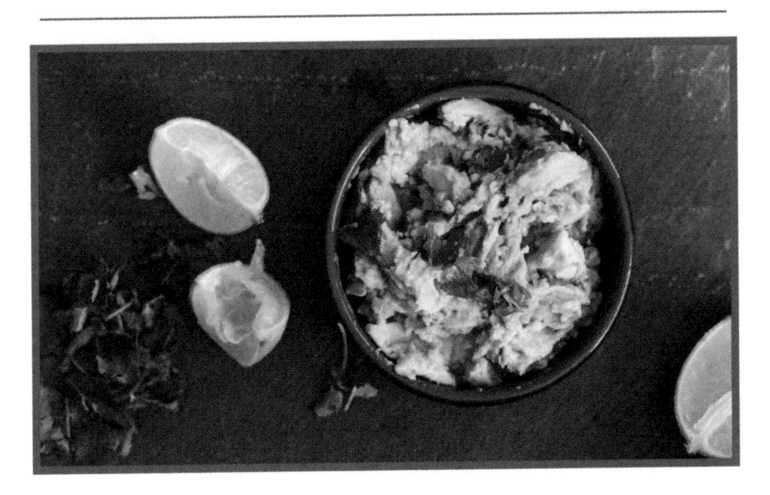

Mix avocado and your favorite guacamole ingredients with these essential oils:

- 1–2 drops Lime
- 1 drop Cilantro

Infused Water

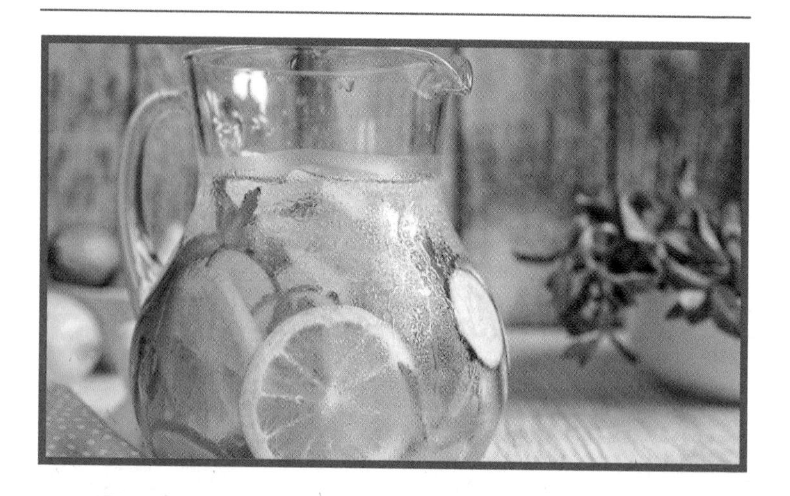

Kick up the flavor in your drinking water by adding citrus essential oils to your glass every morning! While everyone's taste buds are different, I love adding a drop each of the different citrus essential oils:

- **Lemon**
- **Wild Orange**
- **Grapefruit**
- **Lime**

When you're traveling, Grapefruit is the best! It's super detoxifying and helps move those fluids through your body. Fill up a glass (or water bottle) with water and ice and load in those oils! I highly recommend starting with one or two of the citrus oils, then start mixing and matching until you find the mix that's perfect for you.

Cilantro Lime Rice

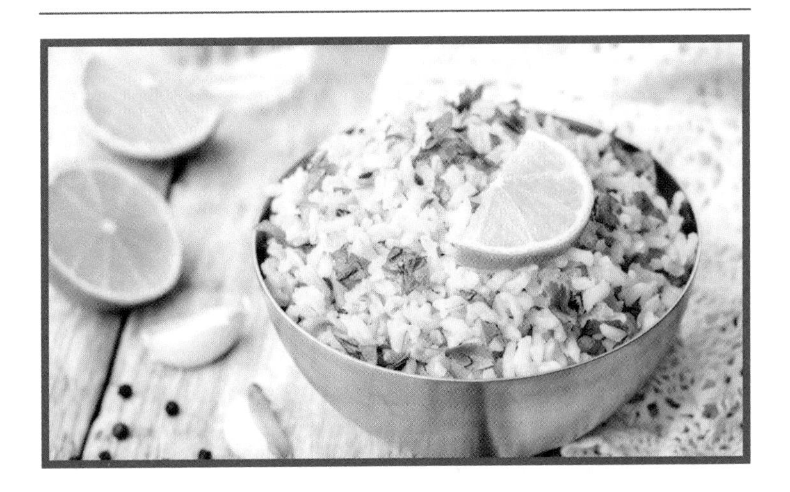

This recipe calls for Lime essential oil, but if you're feeling ambitious you could add some Cilantro oil as well!

Ingredients:

- 1 cup Prepared Rice (White or Brown)
- 2 tbsp. Extra Virgin Olive Oil
- 1 Small Onion
- 2 Cloves Garlic, Finely Diced
- 1 Bunch Cilantro, Chopped or Minced
- 6-8 drops Lime Oil

Instructions:

1. Heat 1 tbsp. Olive Oil in a small skillet.
2. Sautée onion until tender.
3. Add Garlic and cook additional minute or two.
4. In a large bowl, combine:
5. The rest of the olive oil;
6. The onion mixture;

7. Cilantro and Lime essential oils.
8. Spread over rice and mix in.

Marinara Sauce

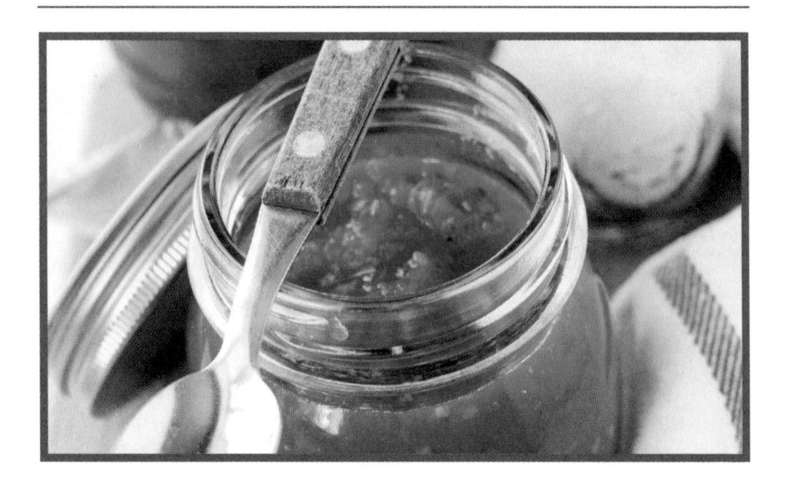

Are you a pasta lover? This marinara sauce, infused with essential oils is both luscious and healthy.

Ingredients:

- 2 pounds Roma Tomatoes, cut in half
- 1 Sliced Onion
- 4 Garlic Cloves
- Olive Oil
- Sea Salt
- Pepper
- 1 drop Basil essential oil
- 1 toothpick Oregano essential oil

Instructions:

Simmer until desired doneness and smother pasta or steamed veggies.

Ginger Peanut Butter Cookies

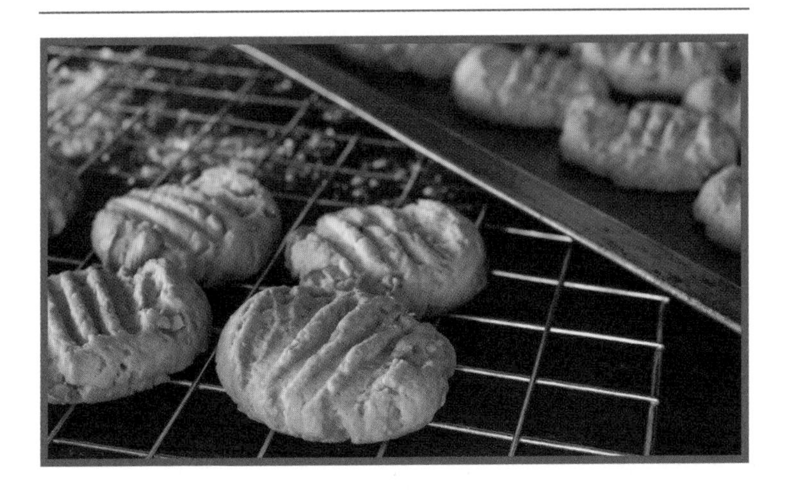

Ingredients:

- 1 cup Peanut Butter
- 1 cup Sugar
- 1 Large Egg or Egg Substitute
- 1 tsp. Vanilla Extract
- 3 drops Ginger essential oil

Instructions:

1. Mix in a large bowl until combined. Shape dough into 1-inch balls.
2. Place balls 1 inch apart on ungreased baking sheets.
3. Flatten gently with tines of a fork.

4. Bake at 325°F for 15 minutes or until golden brown. Delish.

And if you're vegan like me, you have choices!

Vegan Peanut Butter Cookies

Ingredients:

- 1 cup Natural, Unsalted Peanut Butter
- ¼ cup plus 1 tsp. Real Maple Syrup
- 1 tsp Sea Salt
- 1 drop Wild Orange or Cinnamon essential oil (optional)

Instructions:

1. Preheat oven to 350°F. Combine ingredients in food processor.
2. Form into small balls onto lined baking sheet and flatten with a fork. Bake 10 minutes.

Vegan Shish Kabob

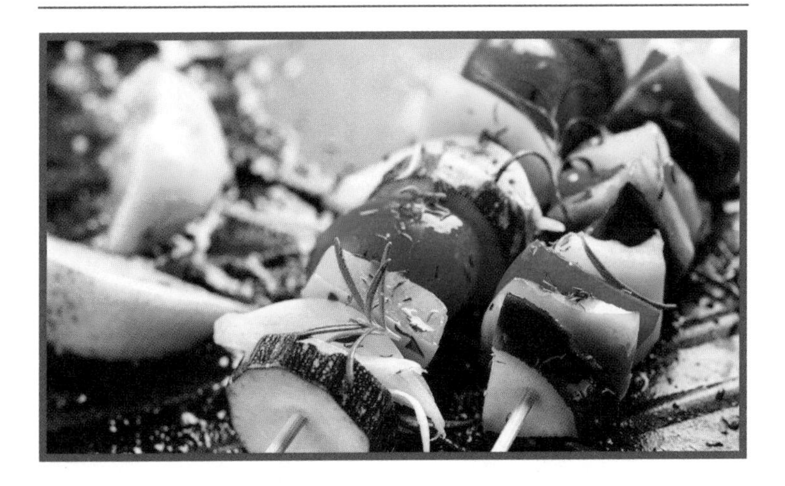

This is one of my favorite meals to cook. It's great because it's vegan, and you can cook these on an indoor grill and stay away from the cold!

Ingredients:

- 2 Zucchini
- 1 package Cherry Tomatoes
- 2 Red Onions
- Yellow and Orange Bell Peppers
- Mushrooms
- Olive Oil
- Cilantro essential oil
- Lime essential oil

Instructions:

1. Chop vegetables into cubes (except mushrooms and tomatoes), toss lightly with olive oil and a pinch of salt and freshly ground pepper.

2. Load the cubes onto skewers; grill lightly to maintain some crunch.
3. Take off skewers, put into a bowl then toss in olive oil with one drop each of Cilantro and Lime essential oil.

Fennel Salad

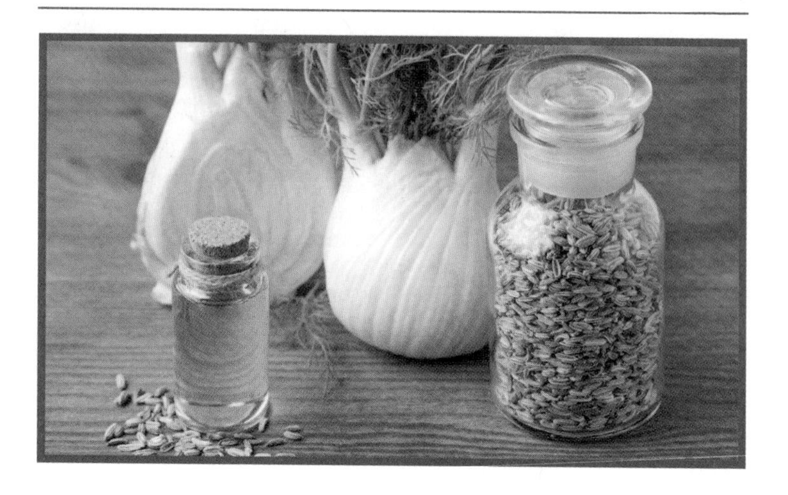

Ingredients:

- 5 oz. Arugula
- 1 small Fennel Bulb, sliced thin
- 2 tbsp. Extra Virgin Olive Oil
- 1 tsp. Lemon zest
- Juice of 1 Lemon
- 2–3 drops Fennel essential oil
- Black Pepper essential oil to taste
- ¼ tsp. Salt

Your Personal Relationship with Oils

Your relationship with essential oils will be what you make of it. Some people have a few favorites and that's all they use. However, I have found it to be the opposite. Most people I've met who try them can't get enough.

Continue to learn and experiment as you go. Trust your intuition to draw you to the oils you need for balance. Don't necessarily go by the scents you like best. Certain oils may smell unpleasant, but surprisingly, they can change your life.

Keep a Journal

Learn as you go and keep an essential oils journal, at least in the beginning. In the journal you can track how you're feeling physically, and also what you're dealing with emotionally and mentally.

Be sure to write down the oils you use and any results you notice when using them.

Life is about choices. Someone doesn't hand us a triptik, a slap on the back, and tell us to "Go for it!" We choose where we go, what we do, and who will accompany us on our journeys. Each choice, whether conscious or unconscious, leads us in a specific direction.

Does that mean we should agonize over making choices? No, because even what we might call bad choices have value, as long as we are willing to get the lesson. Besides, we can un-choose whenever we want.

No matter how challenging, you will ultimately be grateful for the paths you've taken and the choices you've made. I know I am—even the ones that didn't turn out as expected. All of your choices will teach you something about yourself.

The choice I am most grateful for is the choice to live a holistic lifestyle. Because of it, I am healthier and more content, and so is my family. I'm truly living the life I always dreamed of. A whole and happy life is more meaningful if we share it with others. So as a coach, my goal is to empower others to thrive; to be well and happy, too.

That's why I wrote this book. For you.

I want to help YOU become the best possible WHOLE version of yourself. Along with eating healthy foods, exercising, and mental and emotional wellness practices, essential oils are a big part of that.

If I may leave you with something else; I'd like to say this: learn all you can about life and love and most importantly, listen to and trust your own inner knowing. Resist the temptation to look outside yourself for fulfillment.

All the answers you seek are inside. Trust your intuition.

XO,
Hayley

JOURNALING

About the Author

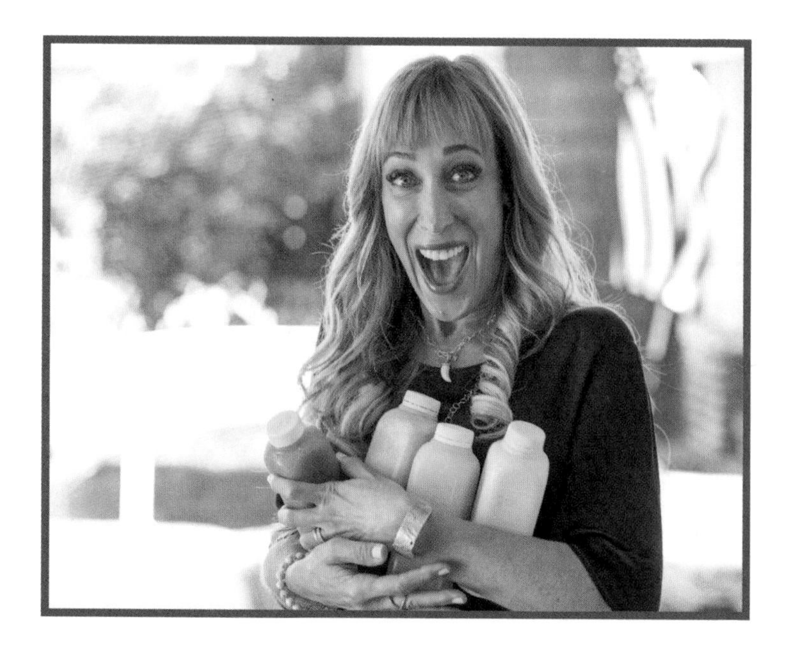

Hayley Hobson is an internationally known author and inspirational speaker. Her podcast, *Hayley Hobson's Whole You*, launched in 2017.

As a life coach, she passionately empowers others to create lifestyle transformations by supporting them in becoming the best possible WHOLE versions of themselves.

Whether at home in the mountains of Boulder, CO or relaxing at her beach house in Cardiff by the Sea, CA, Hayley enjoys spending time with her husband, former world-ranked professional triathlete, Wes Hobson, and their two daughters, Makenna and Madeline. Her vegan lifestyle incorporates juicing, fitness, and spirituality.

In addition to Hayley's coaching programs and online courses, she is a sought-after speaker at global business events. Her programs, presented in more than fifty countries, weave together life coaching principles with strategic business practices. Hayley teaches by consciously monitoring our thoughts, we are in control of the results we are looking for in our personal or business lives.

As a Wellness Advocate, Hayley is credited with achieving the highest ranks in her company in the least amount of time. Today she holds the highest rank of Double Presidential Diamond.

Hayley is an influence among an expanding network of peers and she remains one of the top earners in her company. Her main charitable focus is the building of an orphanage in Haiti that when complete will house up to twenty-five children.

Hayley Hobson has been featured in *The Network Marketing Times, The Four Year Career, Natural Health Magazine, Triathlete Magazine and Mindbodygreen.* She regularly blogs for *Positively Positive* and her social media following exceeds hundreds of thousands. Look for Hayley on Instagram (@HayleyHobson) and Facebook at (https://www.facebook.com/hayleyhobsonwholeyou/).